BREAD MACHINE COOKBOOK

Perfect For The Beginner Baker with Quick and Easy Recipes for Homemade Bread | WOW Family and Friends With Your Baking Creations Including Gluten-Free, Low-Carb Choices & More

By

Beth Anderson Pot

© Copyright 2020 - All rights reserved.

The content contained within this book may not be reproduced, duplicated or transmitted without direct written permission from the author or the publisher. Under no circumstances will any blame or legal responsibility be held against the publisher, or author, for any damages, reparation, or monetary loss due to the information contained within this book. Either directly or indirectly.

Legal Notice:

This book is copyright protected. This book is only for personal use. You cannot amend, distribute, sell, use, quote or paraphrase any part, or the content within this book, without the consent of the author or publisher.

Disclaimer Notice:

Please note the information contained within this document is for educational and entertainment purposes only. All effort has been executed to present accurate, up to date, and reliable, complete information. No warranties of any kind are declared or implied. Readers acknowledge that the author is not engaging in the rendering of legal, financial, medical or professional advice. The content within this book has been derived from various sources. Please consult a licensed professional before attempting any techniques outlined in this book.

By reading this document, the reader agrees that under no circumstances is the author responsible for any losses, direct or indirect, which are incurred as a result of the use of information contained within this document, including, but not limited to, — errors, omissions, or inaccuracies.

Table of Contents

Introduction

Chapter 1. Getting To Know Your Bread Machine

Keeping It Clean

Chapter 2. Bread Machine Cycles

Chapter 3. Art of Selecting and Measuring Ingredients

Chapter 4. Troubleshooting

Benefits Of Using Bread Machine:

Chapter 5. When you're New in Baking Tips: What Can You Do?

The List Of Groceries For The Bread Recipe

Chapter 6. Cheese Breads

1. Onion, Garlic, Cheese Bread
2. Cream Cheese Bread
3. Mozzarella Cheese and Salami Loaf
4. Olive and Cheddar Loaf
5. Cottage Cheese Bread
6. Green Cheese Bread
7. Cheesy Chipotle Bread
8. Cheddar Cheese Basil Bread
9. Olive Cheese Bread
10. Double Cheese Bread
11. Chile Cheese Bacon Bread
12. Blue Cheese Onion Bread
13. Cheddar Sausage Muffins
14. Garlic Bread

15. Feta Oregano Bread
16. Bacon Bread
17. Mozzarella Herbs Bread
18. Cheesy Low Carb Butter & Garlic Bread
19. Low-carb Bagel
20. Cheese & Fruit Stuffed Panini

Chapter 7. Vegetable Breads
21. Beetroot Bread
22. Yeasted Carrot Bread
23. Basil Tomato Bread
24. Savory Onion Bread
25. Confetti Bread
26. Honey Potato Flakes Bread
27. Pretty Borscht Bread
28. Hot Red Pepper Bread
29. French Onion Bread
30. Garlic Onion Pepper Bread
31. Healthy Banana Bread
32. Mushroom Leek Bread
33. Greek Olive Cheese Bread
35. Garden Vegetable Bread
36. Potato Bread
37. Carrot Coriander Bread
38. Perfect Sweet Potato Bread
39. Potato Dill Bread

40. Healthy Celery Loaf

Chapter 8. Gluten Free Bread

41. Gluten-Free Potato Bread
42. Sorghum Bread Recipe
43. Gluten-Free Simple Sandwich Bread
44. Gluten-Free Oat & Honey Bread
45. Gluten-Free Cinnamon Raisin Bread
46. Grain-Free Chia Bread
47. Gluten-Free Pizza Crust
48. Gluten-Free Whole Grain Bread
49. Gluten-Free Pull-Apart Rolls
50. Classic Gluten-Free Bread
51. Gluten-Free Chocolate Zucchini Bread
52. Honey Oat Bread
53. Nutty Cinnamon Bread
54. Nisus Bread
55. Maple Syrup Spice Bread
56. Cherry-Blueberry Loaf
57. Gluten-Free Loaf
58. Healthy Grain-Free Bagels
59. Cream of Orange Bread
60. Gluten-Free Crusty Boule Bread

Chapter 9. Sourdough Breads

61. Sourdough Starter
62. Garlic And Herb Flatbread Sourdough

63. Dinner Rolls
64. Sourdough Boule
65. Herbed Baguette
66. Pumpernickel Bread
67. Sauerkraut Rye
68. Crusty Sourdough Bread
69. Honey Sourdough Bread
70. Multigrain Sourdough Bread
71. Everyday Sourdough Bread
72. Cracked Wheat Bread
73. Pumpkin Spice Sourdough Loaf
74. Sourdough Bread Sticks
75. Cheddar Sourdough Bread
76. Spicy Cheddar Sourdough Bread
77. Beer And Rye Sourdough Bread
78. Blueberry And Lemon Sourdough Bread

Chapter 10. Spice & Herb Breads

79. Original Italian Herb Bread
80. Cinnamon & Dried Fruits Bread
81. Herbal Garlic Cream Cheese Delight
82. Oregano Monza -Cheese Bread
83. Potato Rosemary Loaf
84. Pistachio Cherry Bread
85. Inspiring Cinnamon Bread
86. Lavender Buttermilk Bread

87. Cardamom Cranberry Bread

88. Sesame French Bread

89. Zucchini Bread

90. Banana Split Loaf

91. Cranberry Orange Pecan Bread

92. Caramelized Onion Bread

93. Romano Oregano Bread

94. Parsley Garlic Bread

95. Swiss Olive Bread

96. Super Spice Bread

97. Anise Honey Bread

98. Basic Pecan Bread

Chapter 11. Nut Breads

99. Cranberry Walnut Wheat Bread

100. Brown Sugar Date Nut Swirl Bread

101. Raisin Bread

102. Multigrain Bread

103. Toasted Pecan Bread

104. Market Seed Bread

107. Hazelnut Honey Bread

108. Double Coconut Bread

109. Flax And Sunflower Seed Bread

110. Honey And Flaxseed Bread

111. Pumpkin And Sunflower Seed Bread

112. Seven Grain Bread

113. Wheat Bread With Flax Seed

114. High Fiber Bread

115. High Flavor Bran Head

116. High Protein Bread

117. Whole Wheat Bread With Sesame Seeds

118. Bagels With Poppy Seeds

119. Macadamia Nut Bread

120. Paled Coconut Bread

Chapter 12. Sweet & Chocolate Bread

121. Currant Bread

122. Pineapple Juice Bread

123. Mocha Bread

124. Maple Syrup Bread

125. Peanut Butter & Jelly Bread

126. Brown & White Sugar Bread

127. Molasses Bread

128. Chocolate Zucchini Bread

129. Pumpkin Bread

130. Strawberry Bread

131. Blueberry Bread Loaf

132. Cranberry And Orange Bread

133. Chocolate Chip Beloved Bread

134. Poppy Seed And Prune Bread

135. Blessed Bread

136. Fast And Fabulous

137. Regal Raisin Bread

138. Holiday Holler

139. Charming Challah

140. Chocolate Bread With Hazelnuts

Chapter 13. Whole Wheat Bread

141. Whole Wheat Peanut Butter And Jelly Bread

142. Bread Machine Ezekiel Bread

143. Bread Machine Honey-Oat-Wheat Bread

144. Butter Honey Wheat Bread

145. Buttermilk Bread I

146. Buttermilk Wheat Bread

147. Ricotta & Chive Loaf

148. Crunchy Honey Wheat Bread

149. Easy Whole Wheat Bread

150. Essene Bread For The Bread Machine

151. Hot Buttered Rum Bread

152. Honey-Flavored Bread

153. Pantone Bread

154. Delicious Flax Honey Loaf

155. Raisin Bran Bread

156. Oat Bran Molasses Bread

157. Bran Bread

158. Whole-Wheat Challah

159. Whole-Wheat Sourdough Bread

160. Faithful Italian Semolina Bread

Conclusion

Introduction

Bread Machines have been around for quite some time now. In our early days, they used to be quite a luxury to have in the home. My earliest childhood memory of a bread maker was my mother telling me the aroma of freshly baked bread was making her go crazy and that she was going to take a walk until it cooled down. I don't know when it was exactly but I'm sure it was after the kids were born. That is something all parents have in common. When your kids are young, you don't have anything better to do with yourself than to spend as much time with them as possible. This usually means all day every day. By the time they got to G.G. (those years when they graduate and go out on their own), they were usually exhausted and happy to see the days go by as quickly as the weeks. As we approached our career years we were willing to do anything we could to pass the time as quickly as we possibly could, just so we had a few more precious years left to spend with our children.

Your bread machine is capable of much more than you might have initially suspected. In simple terms, your bread maker is just a basic kitchen appliance that reshapes dough into edible meals. This process is done with the help of a little robot inside your machine. All you have to do is position the ingredients inside of your bread machine correctly and in a timely manner, and the little bot will do the rest of the work for you. The entire process is done in a way that will make your experience in your kitchen much more enjoyable. The main idea behind the bread machine is to make the user's life easier. You, the user, are capable of creating perfect yeast breads, no matter how mundane or exotic, in the same amount of time that it would take you to make normal bread. Your bread maker will make everything as if you are a master baker. It can also make you a variety of different types of bread that could satisfy any feast. The most amazing part about this little gadget is that it is capable of turning your favorite baked goods into a convenient and easy to prepare meal for the entire family. Those recipes that you have spent hours perfecting are now waiting patiently for you in your bread maker, ready to be baked. The whole process can be done in a matter of hours, making it possible to fit a whole week's worth of meals into your schedule. The main purpose of using a bread maker is to create delicious treats that would otherwise require tons of daily effort. The whole process of bread making is actually a lot quicker than many expect. Due to the highly developed technology that has been invested in the bread machine, it is now capable of outperforming many professional bakers in terms of the amount of food it can produce. Your bread maker does not skimp on the quality of the ingredients that were used to create your meals. A bread maker can make your meals in a matter of hours. The whole process allows you to set a timer and forget about it. This kitchen appliance can check on the status of your dough every two hours, in case you choose to check up on it. As long as you keep with the instructions that were given to you along with your bread maker, you will be very happy with the results. The bread machine is capable of producing much more than just soft bread. You can also make hearty bread perfect for breakfast. The same machine can also make pizza dough, pasta and cinnamon buns. If it can be baked, it can be created in the bread maker. The technology used in your bread machine will have you logging tons of hours of leisure time in your kitchen.

Using a bread machine to make bread is much simpler than you may initially think. Follow the exceptional bread-making instructions that were given to you. This will ensure that your unit runs smoothly. The purpose of this is to ensure that you have the best baking experience possible. This is a process, you are going to enjoy. Not only will you be able to spend more time with your loved ones but you will also be able to create a variety of different breads to fit all of your family's tastes. Before you know it, you will be addicted to making bread in the bread maker. Your machine is capable of only making the most delicious meals. Although there are many machines out there, the ones created by Lee Stafford Company are the ones you need to invest your hard-earned money. The bread machine is capable of making a variety of different types of meals. The only thing you will need to do is purchase a bread machine. Your machine is capable of turning your favorite meals into a soft, delicious meal that is also extremely nutritious.

Accessories for bread machine

There are a lot of accessories that can make bread-making much easier. You should know that a bread maker is not a single machine. It's more like a cooking range with a lot of different attachments. Here are some important accessories for bread makers, which will help you make successful bread.

The first thing you will need is a recipe book. This cookbook will provide you with a wide range of recipes for different types of bread, even for pizza dough or homemade pasta. You will need a recipe book in order to make something tasty.

The second one is a measuring cup. It will help you make the dough in the right amount.

And the accessory that is most important, bread pan. A bread pan is a container, which you put the dough in and the bread maker will do the rest of the work.

Guide for the first time

In case this is your first time using a bread maker, you should read this guide. You have to find a good recipe book, create your own recipe or just use a recipe that is provided in the bread maker cookbook.

Be sure that you always prepare the recipe properly. If you don't prepare the recipe right, the result will be disappointing.

Chapter 1.   Getting To Know Your Bread Machine

There are a few things you will want to do before you start baking. First and foremost get acquainted with your machine. After all, it's an important piece of electronic equipment in your kitchen. You will want to read the owner's manual thoroughly and keep it handy to refer to often. It will tell you everything about the machine and the cycles. You can even find recipes for every cycle including their settings. As well, there is a booklet which comes with the machine that gives you tips on using the machine and giving your bread its best taste and texture.

Getting acquainted with the cycle settings with your bread machine is a good habit to get into. You will want to select your cycle depending upon what you are making. The cycle settings of bread machines vary from machine to machine. Once you get used to your machine you will probably find that there is more than one cycle that will make the task easier to accomplish. For instance, there is a cycle to make regular loaves of bread. Some machines have a stretch cycle, which is a programmable thermostat within the machine that gives you a quicker cycle. It is best when you are in a rush. Your bread machine will tell you the time it requires for each cycle.

Keeping It Clean

Proper cleaning should be done every time you use the machine. You will also want to do regular cleaning every month. Here are some steps to follow:

Clean the bread pan and the kneading blade. You will be able to remove the kneading blade while it is still attached to the pan. Place the kneading blade in the dishwasher. Wash the bread pan by hand. After you have finished making the bread remove the bread pan from the machine and wipe a damp paper towel over the kneading blade and the pan. The kneading blade should be damp so you will not scratch the machine. Pay special attention to the side that contacts the pan so that it does not become dull. Allow the blade to air dry. Do not allow the bread pan rack to dry or get in contact with plastic. Clean the bread maker lid and the control panel. Scrub them with a very damp paper towel. Wipe the interior parts of the machine. There should be a small lamp near the clock. It's a light that you will notice until you clean it. Do not clean the metal surface of the clock. You will never know if it has been used. There should be a light across the front of the machine. It's the indicator light. Never use abrasive material that you can find in your kitchen such as steel wool.

Make sure that you get the entire residue from the bread pan. You will want to make sure that you do not leave residue in the machine. It could affect the taste of your food.

On a regular cleaning cycle be sure to clean the machine. Add one cup of white vinegar to one of water and place the machine on a regular cycle. Wipe all the interior parts of the machine. Give the kneading blade a thorough wash and let it air dry in the machine.

Also, you will want to spray the kneading blade with a new coat of nonstick cooking spray. You should be able to either replace the kneading blade or replace part of the machine. Some people buy a combination of both. You will never know which one will get damaged first.

Chapter 2.   Bread Machine Cycles

The bread machine cycle is a turning and kneading cycle. You knead the dough that passes through the machine using the kneading action. One cycle of bread baking can only give you one loaf of bread. Sometimes, you will want a bun or something of this nature. So, now you will have to add a cycle for that or use a bread maker for multiple purposes.

Also, you can use a water bath or steam cycle. Some machines will tell you what cycles you have available for some types of bread and they don't tell you what you can do with the bread maker. You will want to know what you can use your bread maker for. There are many different uses for the bread maker that you will find to be useful to you. If your bread maker tells you everything about its cycles, read the cycles and find out what you can do with your machine. Especially the ones you will use often.

Your bread will look and taste good if you follow the cycles that the bread maker gives you. However you will know best how you like your bread in a particular cycle. Bread maker machines vary from one another. You should read the manual that came with your machine to learn more about the different cycles.

Making bread is not a difficult process. If you take your time and follow the instructions in the instructions that came with the bread maker that you have recently purchased then you will be a master baker in no time.

1. Basic Cycle: A program that will bake a loaf of bread for you with or without raising agent (yeast). With the Basic Cycle, there are no options for change.
2. Whole-wheat Cycle: If you would like to utilize whole-grain flour, this is a great choice for you. The whole-wheat cycle will help you add the missing fiber and nutrients into your bread and it will also make it fresher for longer periods of time.
3. Quick/Rapid Cycle: Best used for mixing and kneading bread dough.
4. Dough Cycle: A program that will knead the ingredients (flour and water) into a nice smooth dough. If you are making bread, this is a great choice.

5. Sweet bread Cycle: A program that will make bread with high sugar content.
6. Nut or Raisin Cycle: A program that will knead nuts and raisins into the dough during the mixing process.
7. French bread Cycle: A program that will make a loaf of that tender French bread that tastes so good, in the humidity of your own home.
8. Quick Bread Cycle: Similar to the Dough Cycle but will use a bit more water.
9. Jam Cycle: A program that allows you to make jams by the cup.
10. Cake Cycle: A program that you can put cake batter into the machine and choose different cake batter recipes from the manual included with the machine. Cake batters can include but are not limited to chocolate cake batter, yellow cake batter, and more.
11. Fruit and Nut Cycle: A program that will take the dry ingredients and mix them in with the wet ingredients and bake bread that is full of fruits, nuts, and grains.
12. Vegetable Cycle: A program that will bake bread with vegetables.
13. Fast Bake Cycle: Depending on the machine you can choose a rapid bake cycle to make bread in less than ninety minutes and that still tastes fresh.
14. Bake cycle: A program that will bake bread in the oven inside the machine.

Chapter 3.   Art of Selecting and Measuring Ingredients

In order to achieve great results every time you use your bread machine, the art of selection and measuring ingredients is of the utmost importance. It may seem like a lot to remember but once you do it a couple of times, it will be a breeze to do every time. Before you get started, make sure that you have all of the ingredients and tools that you will need in order to complete the recipe you are working on. The obvious items are flour, salt, water, and yeast. You should also have room in your freezer for the Ziploc bag that you will be used to store the bread once it is baked. Don't forget the bread maker. Also, don't forget your measuring cup. It is important to have one that can measure at a precise level so that you do not accidentally add too much flour or salt to the machine recipe and end up with bad-tasting bread. You also want to make sure that you have all of your ingredients measured out. One-half cup of flour is not necessarily the same as one-half cup of water. Not all flour is the same, so it is very important that you try to measure the flour as accurately as possible. For example, if you accidentally use a cup of flour that reads a little more than half a cup, then the flour that you need to use and the amount of water that you need to add could be touchy. Once you have the ingredients measured out, all you need to do is to plug it in and follow the instructions that come with the machine.

There are many things that can go wrong if you do not measure ingredients accurately every time that you make your bread machine recipe. First of all, you will not have properly textured bread if you do not measure the ingredients properly. Also, if you measure uneven ingredients, then you will have a baking disaster.

What you need to remember is that the best results will be achieved when following the recipe exactly. Feel free to save your inspiration you may have for future recipes but just use the same ingredients. Here is a list of items you should always have on hand in your refrigerator:

1. High-quality bread flour: Bread flour should be labeled as "bread flour". The label should be stamped on the top right-hand part of the flour container.

All but the finest flour may have an additive. The words "high protein flour" is not a good choice because it does not taste right in bread.
2. Flour: Many bakers like to use their own flour but no matter how good the flour is, it is still just bread flour.
3. Sugar: The proper amount of sugar should be about 1/3 of the water. One cup should be enough sugar for two loaves and 1/3 cup is just right for one loaf of bread.
4. Yeast: You need to use the fresh package of plain flour yeast. Do not try to use the packets of quick or rapid rise yeast. They will give you a false rise and tough dough.
5. Yeast - regular and quick: The best idea is to get yeast in bulk and store it in the freezer until used. Make sure to check the expiration date if you don't intend to use your yeast within two weeks.
6. Salt: A good quality salt is a must in the breading process. Use "iodized table salt" in all your measurements.
7. Unsalted butter: Plain, soft, unsalted butter is a must in any bread recipe.
8. Milk/water: For baking purposes use milk with up to 4.5%. Do not use skim milk.
9. Butter - softened: This should be a soft and smooth butter. Before using the butter, make sure it is room temperature, free of any wax and that it is flowing freely.
10. Eggs: The eggs are used to help the bread rise. A little extra to this recipe can make a huge difference in the quality of the bread. In this recipe you can even use an egg substitute.
11. Evaporated Milk: Evaporated milk is a great item to add to bread recipes. It will add a special flavor and add a little sweetness to it. This item is usually found in the canned food aisle near the biscuits. The brand does not matter too much. As long as it is #1 you should be good to go.

Chapter 4.   Troubleshooting

1. Not enough water: If the dough did not seem to be doing as it should, then you can try adding a bit more water. You may have added more flour than you need. Do not add any more flour when you're kneading in the dough. The dough will feel stiff at first. That's the way it should be.
2. Too much water: If the dough seems too wet and does not get to the kneading stage, then you will need to add extra flour during the kneading process. You will need to add flour about ¼ cups at a time.
3. Dense and short rise: If your bread did not rise to the top of the pan during the initial baking cycle, then try rolling the dough out on the counter. Before punching down the dough onto the pan, roll up the dough from the bottom and let it rise to the top. This will give it a denser rise and it should come out perfectly. If that doesn't work you can try to add an additional ½ inch of flour or more.
4. Crust too thick: If the crust seems too thick, then add another tablespoon or so of water. If you add too much water then you will have to add flour. Do not add more than ¼ cup to the recipe at one time.
5. Bread crumbly: If the bread in the loaf pan crumbled out of the pan during the cooling down process, then you can try to mix in some extra flour.
6. Course Texture: If you think you have added too much flour, then add more water.
7. Loaf Shaped Wrong: The loaf may have risen larger in one direction than the other. You can use a bread knife to cut the loaf into a perfect shape just before baking. For most people it really doesn't matter if your bread is not perfectly shaped. The taste will still be great.
8. Gummy Texture: If you find that your bread did not rise or if the bread did not have a pleasant flavor, then you may have used skim milk instead of regular milk.

Benefits Of Using Bread Machine:

1. The bread machine program is designed to be foolproof. Even a beginner with little time can learn how to use it in just a few instructions.
2. The recipes are often healthier and cause less caloric intake than other recipes.
3. Even though the recipes are easier to follow, the taste will be just as good as home-baked bread.
4. No matter if you're at home or you're on vacation, you can make fresh bread in just a few minutes.
5. The bread machine is not bulky like your conventional oven and it can easily fit in almost any small kitchen space.
6. It's the perfect mode if you have a large family and you want a low maintenance machine. Have fresh bread whenever you want with very little work.

Eight Reasons Why You Should Bake Your Own Bread in a Bread Machine:

1. Convenience: Baking bread in a bread machine takes less time than making bread at home. The ingredients are already measured and everything is measured on the fly.
2. Equity: Baking bread at home can take very long. You have to measure the flour right before you start baking. Measuring with a cup can take almost 10 minutes. With a bread maker, the ingredients are already measured and labeled on the bread pan.
3. Taste: When you do use a bread machine though, you will finally be able to enjoy homemade fresh baked bread. You will feel the hot bread right out of the machine while the fresh smell of the bread will attract all the family members.
4. Health: Baking bread in a bread machine lowers the glycemic index. The grain bread you get in a bread maker reduces the fat content and the number of calories consumed by a very significant amount.
5. Baked Bread: A lot of times slow-baked bread can result in poorer texture and taste. If you are looking for faster bread, then baking bread in a bread maker is not for you.

6. Equipment: Baking bread in a bread machine will save a lot of space in your kitchen. Packed items are not always the best choice. More space means that you can use a better quality pan that can make.
7. Cleanup: Baking bread in a bread machine will make it easier for you to clean up. The bread machine pan is also easy to clean.
8. Recipes: You can also find bread machine recipes for cookies, cakes and even dinners.

Chapter 5.   When you're New in Baking Tips: What Can You Do?

Your yeast will bubble and get foamy when you add sugar or honey to it. Still be careful that the yeast is not burned or you might ruin the whole **recipe. The** mixture should be warm when you add the yeast to it. The ideal temperature of the mixture for yeast is 75 degrees Fahrenheit. Below this temperature, the yeast will be killed and your bread will not rise at all. You will need something that can measure the temperature of your mixture.

Salt is also vital for your bread to rise. You should also add it to the mixture for even feeding the yeast. Set your bread machine to the "dough" setting. Along with the yeast and salt, you can add 1/2 cup all-purpose flour and 2-1/4 cups of bread maker mix. This will use the machine's basic program for making bread. You can customize your bread machine's settings as well. This will depend on your cooking preferences.

Once you have made your dough, you will need to let it proof. A bread machine will however cause the dough to proof in about 45 minutes. This will enable you to have a ready-made loaf of bread if you need one and will not take up even more time. Also, the dough will ferment faster and better.

You can add some healthy elements to your bread machine bread. For instance, you can add vegetables, fruits and grains to it.

Cereals are ideal for bread machine baking. They absorb water during baking and will add flavor. Try adding in your bread machine:

Try adding some flavors with the banana to the loaf. This will add some cream-cheese-like flavors to your bread.

You can also try adding nuts into the bread mix. Add half in and half even out the oil in prosciutto. This will add some coating to the bread.

Washing the pot before using it only removes germs, not dirt. Instead, use a soft cloth moistened with warm water, and rubs the pot. Or, use the steam/dry cycle of your dishwasher.

Don't be afraid to use a lot of liquid, like milk or water, instead of dry ingredients. Just remember that in the baguettes and other artisan breads for which the execution is not 100% accurate, the bread falls apart...

Wipe the utensil thoroughly and dry well before storing it.

When a recipe calls for toasting, careful, dark bread will be burned more quickly than light bread. It will also burn faster if it is thick. You will have to learn by experience as to how to judge when dark bread has been toasted and when pale bread is perfect for consumption.

The List Of Groceries For The Bread Recipe

Yeast

Powdered milk

Butter

Softened butter

Sugar

Black pepper

Ground cayenne pepper

Honey

Baking is fun. It is accompanied by creativity and passion. Baking is also more than recipes. Baking is about satisfaction, and it is about giving you what you want. Baking is about being with your friends and family. Baking is thus a good experience that will enable you to be a competent baker. Many people join baking class with their friends and their families. There are times when they sing and dancing during the baking class. And they also go a part of the way when they make a cake or cupcakes. And of course, when they make bread, it is a great experience for everybody.

There are also times when they make bread for their family and friends then. One of the things that people love to bake is bread.

Chapter 6.   Cheese Breads

1. Onion, Garlic, Cheese Bread

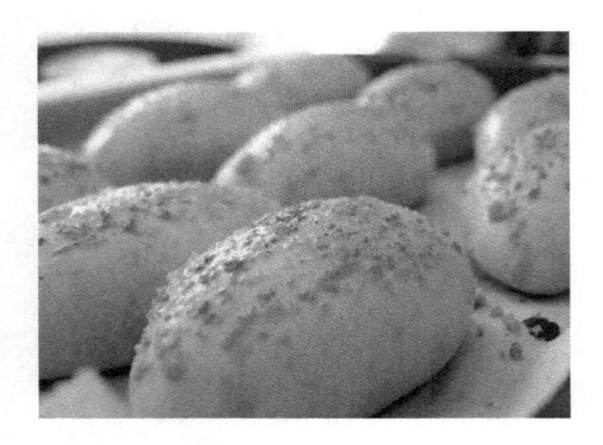

Preparation Time: 50 minutes

Cooking Time: 40 minutes

Servings: One loaf

Ingredients:

- 3 tablespoons dried minced onion
- 3 cups bread flour
- 2 teaspoons Garlic powder
- 2 teaspoons Active dry yeast
- 2 tablespoons White sugar
- 2 tablespoons Margarine
- 2 tablespoons Dry milk powder
- 1 cup shredded sharp cheddar cheese
- 1 1/8 cups warm water
- 1 1/2 teaspoon salt

Directions:

1. In the order suggested by the manufacturer, put the flour, water, powdered milk, margarine or butter, salt, and yeast in the bread pan.
2. Press the basic cycle with a light crust. When the manufacturer directs the sound alerts, add two teaspoons of the onion flakes, the garlic powder, and shredded cheese.
3. After the last kneed, sprinkle the remaining onion flakes over the dough.

Nutrition:

Calories: 204 calories

Total Carbohydrate: 29 g

Total Fat: 6 g

Protein: 8 g

2. Cream Cheese Bread

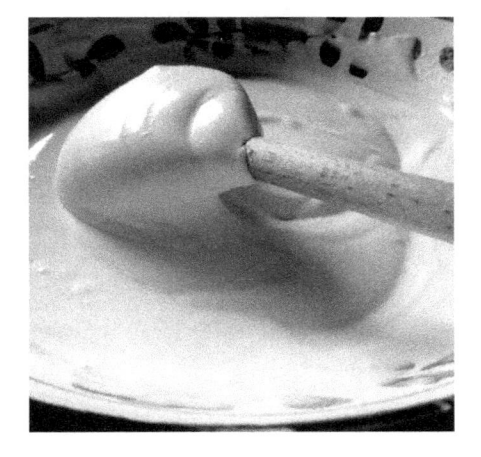

Preparation Time: 60 minutes

Cooking Time: 35 minutes

Servings: 1 loaf

Ingredients:

- 1/2 cup Water
- 1/2 cup Cream
- Cheese softened
- 4 tablespoons melted butter
- 1 Beaten egg
- 4 tablespoons Sugar
- 1 teaspoon salt
- 3 cups bread flour
- 1 1/2 teaspoons Active dry yeast

Directions:

1. Place the ingredients in the pan in order, as suggested by your bread machine.
2. After removing it from a device, please place it in a greased 9x5 loaf pan after the cycle.
3. Cover and let rise until doubled.
4. Bake for approximately 35 minutes

Nutrition:

Calories: 150 calories

Total Carbohydrate: 24 g

Total Fat: 5 g

Protein: 3 g

3. Mozzarella Cheese and Salami Loaf

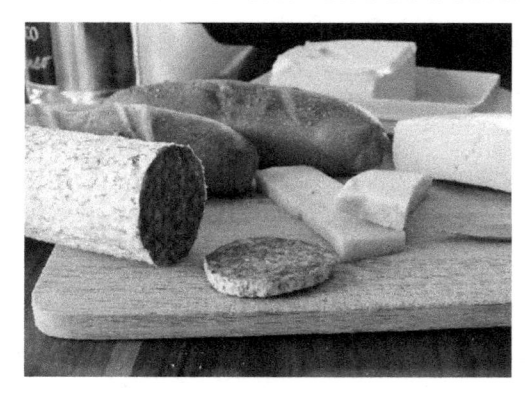

Preparation Time: 2 hours and 50 minutes

Cooking Time: 45 minutes

Servings: 1 loaf

Ingredients:

- ¾ cup water, set at 80 degrees F
- 1/3 cup mozzarella cheese, shredded
- 4 teaspoons sugar
- 2/3 teaspoon salt
- 2/3 teaspoon dried basil
- Pinch of garlic powder
- 2 cups + 2 tablespoons white bread flour
- 1 teaspoon instant yeast
- ½ cup hot salami, finely diced

Directions:

1. Add the listed ingredients to your bread machine (except salami), following the manufactures instructions.
2. Set the bread machine's program to Basic/White Bread and the crust type to light. Press Start.
3. Let the bread machine work and wait until it beeps. It is your indication to add the remaining ingredients at this point, add the salami.
4. Wait until the remaining bake cycle completes.

5. Once the loaf is done, take the bucket out from the bread machine and let it rest for 5 minutes.
6. Gently shake the bucket, remove the loaf, transfer the loaf to a cooling rack, and slice.
7. Serve and enjoy!

Nutrition:

Calories: 164 calories

Total Carbohydrate: 28 g

Total Fat: 3 g

Protein: 6 g

Sugar: 2 g

4. Olive and Cheddar Loaf

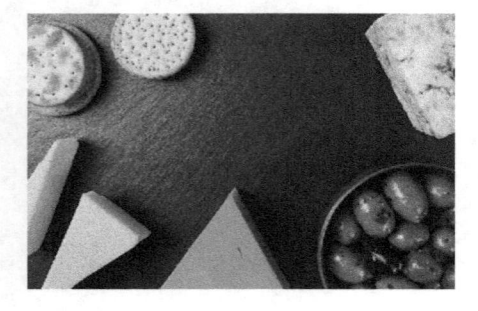

Preparation Time: 2 hours and 50 minutes

Cooking Time: 45 minutes

Servings: 1 loaf

Ingredients:

- 1 cup water, room temperature
- Four teaspoons sugar
- ¾ teaspoon salt

- 1 and 1/ cups sharp cheddar cheese, shredded
- 3 cups bread flour
- Two teaspoons active dry yeast
- ¾ cup pimiento olives, drained and sliced

Directions:

1. Add the listed ingredients to your bread machine (except salami), following the manufactures instructions.
2. Set the bread machine's program to Basic/White Bread and the crust type to Light. Press Start.
3. Let the bread machine work and wait until it beeps. This is your indication to add the remaining ingredients. At this point, add the salami.
4. Wait until the remaining bake cycle completes.
5. Once the loaf is done, take the bucket out from the bread machine and let it rest for 5 minutes.
6. Gently shake the bucket, remove the loaf, transfer the loaf to a cooling rack, and slice.
7. Serve and enjoy!

Nutrition:

Calories: 124 calories

Total Carbohydrate: 19 g

Total Fat: 4 g

Protein: 5 g

Sugar: 5 g

5. Cottage Cheese Bread

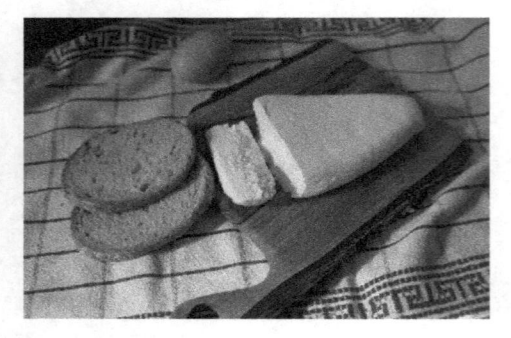

Preparation Time: 2 hours and 50 minutes

Cooking Time: 45 minutes

Servings: 1 loaf

Ingredients:

- 1/2 cup water
- 1 cup cottage cheese
- Two tablespoons margarine
- 1 egg
- 1 tablespoon white sugar
- 1/4 teaspoon baking soda
- 1 teaspoon salt
- 3 cups bread flour
- 2 1/2 teaspoons active dry yeast

Directions:

1. Into the bread machine, place the ingredients according to the ingredients list's order, then push the start button. In case the dough looks too sticky, feel free to use up to half a cup more bread flour.

Nutrition:

Calories: 171 calories

Total Carbohydrate: 26.8 g

Cholesterol: 18 mg

Total Fat: 3.6 g

Protein: 7.3 g

Sodium: 324 mg

6. Green Cheese Bread

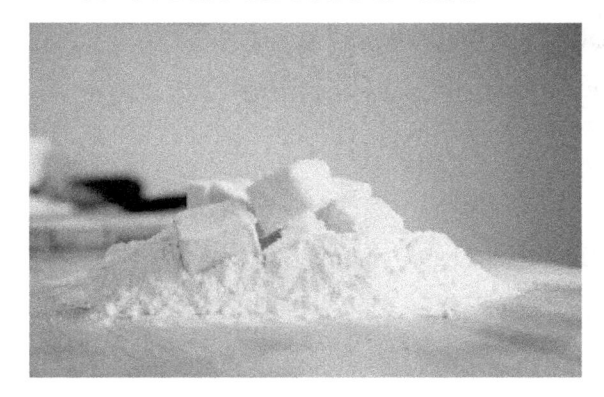

Preparation Time: 3 hours

Cooking Time: 15 minutes

Servings: 8 pcs

Ingredients:

- ¾ cup lukewarm water
- 1 Tablespoon sugar
- 1 teaspoon kosher salt
- 2 Tablespoon green cheese
- 1 cup of wheat bread machine flour
- 9/10 cup whole-grain flour, finely ground
- 1 teaspoon bread machine yeast
- 1 teaspoon ground paprika

Directions:

1. Place all the dry and liquid ingredients, except paprika, in the pan and follow the instructions for your bread machine.
2. Pay particular attention to measuring the ingredients. Use a measuring cup, measuring spoon, and kitchen scales to do so.
3. Dissolve yeast in warm milk with a saucepan and add in the last turn.
4. Add paprika after the beep or place it in the dispenser of the bread machine.
5. Set the baking program to BASIC and the crust type to DARK.
6. If the dough is too wet, adjust the recipe's amount of flour and liquid.
7. When the program has ended, take the pan out of the bread machine and cool for 5 minutes.
8. Shake the loaf out of the pan. If necessary, use a spatula.
9. Wrap the bread with a kitchen towel and set it aside for an hour. Otherwise, you can cool it on a wire rack.

Nutrition:

Calories: 118 calories

Total Carbohydrate: 23.6 g

Cholesterol: 2 g

Total Fat: 1 g

Protein: 4.1 g

Sodium: 304 mg

Sugar: 1.6 g

7. Cheesy Chipotle Bread

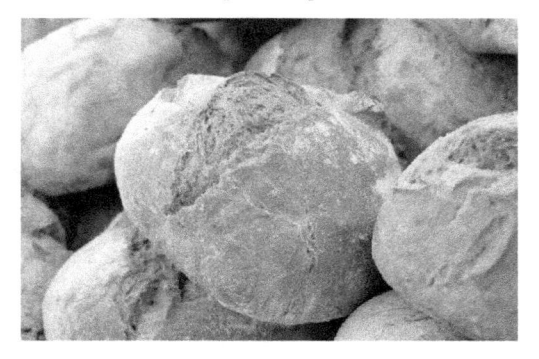

Preparation Time: 2 hours

Cooking Time: 15 minutes

Servings: 8 pcs

Ingredients:

- 2/3 cup water, set at 80°F to 90°F
- 1½ tablespoons sugar
- 1½ tablespoons powdered skim milk
- ¾ teaspoon salt
- ½ teaspoon chipotle chili powder
- 2 cups white bread flour
- ½ cup (2 ounces) shredded sharp Cheddar cheese
- ¾ teaspoon instant yeast

Directions:

1. Place the ingredients in your machine as recommended on it.
2. Make a program on the device for basic white bread, select light or medium crust, and press Start.
3. When the loaf is finished, remove the bucket from the device.
4. Let the loaf cool for a minute.
5. Gently shake the bucket and remove the loaf and turn it out onto a rack to cool.

Nutrition:

Calories: 139 calories

Total Carbohydrate: 27 g

Total Fat: 1g

Protein: 6 g

Sodium: 245 mg

8. Cheddar Cheese Basil Bread

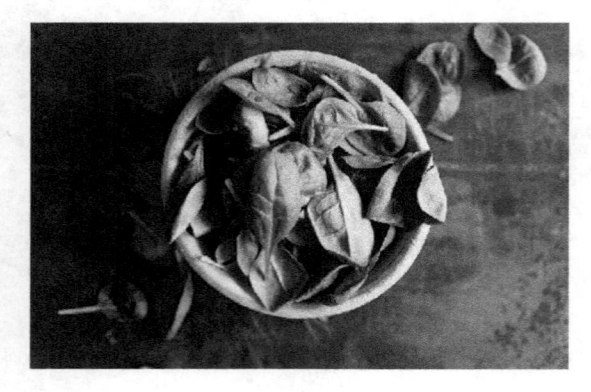

Preparation Time: 2 hours

Cooking Time: 15 minutes

Servings: 8 pcs

Ingredients:

- 2/3 cup milk, set at 80°F to 90°F
- Two teaspoons melted butter, cooled
- Two teaspoons sugar
- 2/3 teaspoon dried basil
- ½ cup (2 ounces) shredded sharp Cheddar cheese
- ½ teaspoon salt
- 2 cups white bread flour

- One teaspoon active dry yeast.

Directions:

1. Place the ingredients in your machine as recommended on it.
2. Make a Program on the machine for basic white Bread, select Light or medium crust, and press Start.
3. When the loaf is finished, remove the bucket from the machine.
4. Let the loaf cool for a minute.
5. Gently shake the bucket and remove the loaf and turn it out onto a rack to cool.

Nutrition:

Calories: 166 calories

Total Carbohydrate: 26 g

Total Fat: 4g

Protein: 6 g

Sodium: 209 mg

9. Olive Cheese Bread

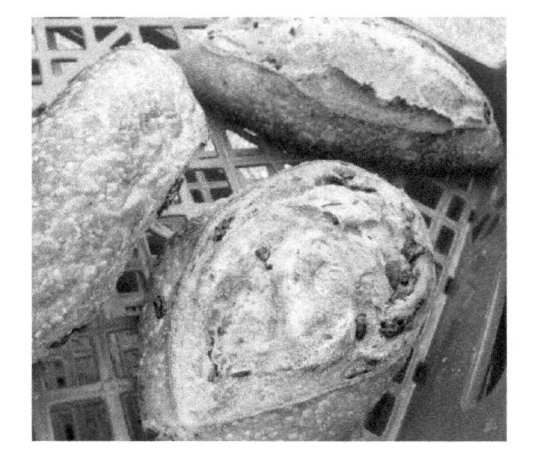

Preparation Time: 2 hours

Cooking Time: 15 minutes

Servings: 8 pcs

Ingredients:

- 2/3 cup milk, set at 80°F to 90°F
- 1 tablespoon melted butter cooled
- 2/3 Teaspoon minced garlic
- 1 tablespoon sugar
- 2/3 teaspoon salt
- 2 cups white bread flour
- ½ cup (2 ounces) shredded Swiss cheese
- ¾ teaspoon bread machine or instant yeast
- ¼ cup chopped black olives

Directions:

1. Place the ingredients in your device as recommended on it.
2. Make a program on the machine for basic white Bread, select Light or medium crust, and press Start.
3. When the loaf is finished, remove the bucket from the machine.
4. Let the loaf cool for a minute.
5. Gently shake the bucket and remove the loaf and turn it out onto a rack to cool.

Nutrition:

Calories: 175 calories

Total Carbohydrate: 27 g

Total Fat: 5g

Protein: 6 g

Sodium: 260 mg

10. Double Cheese Bread

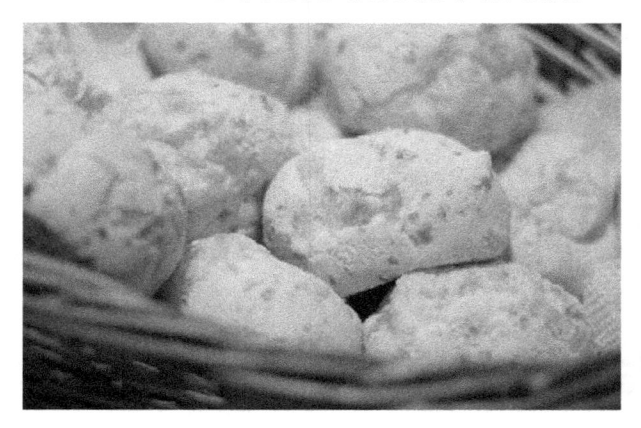

Preparation Time: 2 hours

Cooking Time: 15 minutes

Servings: 8 pcs

Ingredients:

- ¾ cup plus one tablespoon milk, at 80°F to 90°F
- 2 teaspoons butter, melted and cooled
- 4 teaspoons sugar
- 2/3 teaspoon salt
- 1/3 teaspoon freshly ground black pepper
- Pinch cayenne pepper
- 1 cup (4 ounces) shredded aged sharp Cheddar cheese
- 1/3 cup shredded or grated Parmesan cheese
- 2 cups white bread flour
- ¾ teaspoon instant yeast

Directions:

1. Place the ingredients in your machine as recommended on it.
2. Make a program on the device for Basic White bread, select light or medium crust, and press Start.
3. When the loaf is finished, remove the bucket from the device.
4. Let the loaf cool for a minute.

5. Gently shake the bucket and remove the loaf and turn it out onto a rack to cool.

Nutrition:

Calories: 183 calories

Total Carbohydrate: 28 g

Total Fat: 4g

Protein: 6 g

Sodium: 344 mg

11.   Chile Cheese Bacon Bread

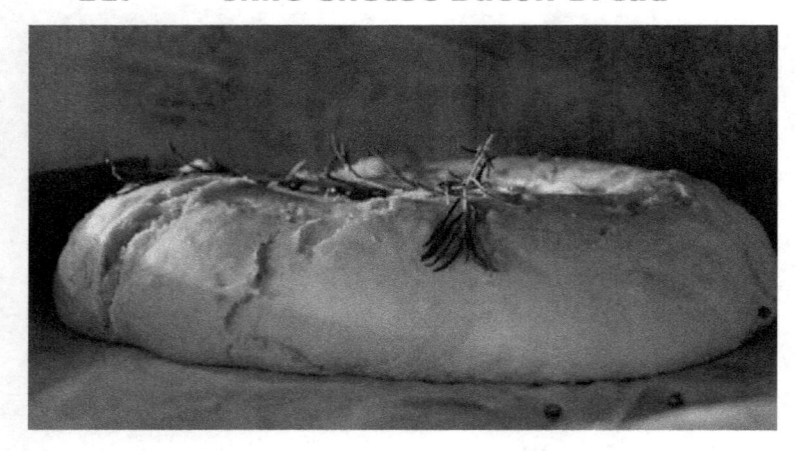

Preparation Time: 2 hours

Cooking Time: 15 minutes

Servings: 8 pcs

Ingredients:

- 1/3 cup milk, set at 80°F to 90°F
- One teaspoon melted butter cooled
- One tablespoon honey

- One teaspoon salt
- 1/3 cup chopped and drained green Chile
- 1/3 cup grated Cheddar cheese
- 1/3 cup chopped cooked bacon
- 2 cups white bread flour
- 1 1/3 teaspoons bread machine or instant yeast

Directions:

1. Place the ingredients in your device as recommended on it.
2. Make a program on the machine for basic white Bread, select Light or medium crust, and press Start.
3. When the loaf is finished, remove the bucket from the device.
4. Let the loaf cool for a minute.
5. Gently shake the bucket and remove the loaf and turn it out onto a rack to cool.

Nutrition:

Calories: 174 calories

Total Carbohydrate: 404 g

Total Fat: 4 g

Protein: 6 g

Sodium: 1 mg

12. **Blue Cheese Onion Bread**

Preparation Time: 2-hours

Cooking Time: 15 Minutes

Servings: 10

Ingredients:

- ½ cup of blue cheese, crumbled
- 1 tsp. unsalted melted butter
- 1 tsp. fresh rosemary, chopped
- 1 ½ cup of fine almond flour
- 3 teaspoons olive oil
- 1 teaspoon baking powder
- ½ cup of warm water
- 1 yellow onion sliced and sautéed in butter until golden brown
- 2 garlic cloves, crushed
- 1 teaspoon Swerve sweetener
- 1 teaspoon salt

Directions:

1. Prepare a mixing container, where you will combine the almond flour, swerve sweetener, baking powder, freshly chopped rosemary, crumbled blue cheese, sautéed sliced onion, salt, and crushed garlic.
2. Get another container to combine the warm water, melted butter, and extra virgin olive oil.
3. As per the instructions in your machine's manual, pour the ingredients into the bread pan, taking care to follow how to mix in the yeast.
4. Place the bread pan in the device, select the basic bread setting, together with the bread size and crust type, if available, then press start once you have closed the machine's lid.
5. When the bread is ready, using oven mitts, remove the bread pan from the device.
6. Use a stainless spatula to extract the bread from the pan, and turn the pan upside down on a metallic rack where the bread will cool off before slicing it.

Nutrition:

Calories 100,

Fat: 6 g,

Carb 3 g,

Protein 11 g.

13. Cheddar Sausage Muffins

Preparation Time: 1-hour

Cooking Time: 25 Minutes

Servings: 8

Ingredients:

- 6 oz. Cooked sausage, grease drained, thinly sliced
- ¼ cup water
- 1 tbsp. baking powder
- ¼ cup heavy cream
- 1 cup shredded sharp white cheddar cheese
- 1 ½ cups almond flour
- ½ tsp. Italian seasoning
- ½ tsp. Sea salt
- 1 tbsp. Chopped fresh chives
- 2 minced large garlic cloves
- 1 large egg
- 4 oz. Softened cream cheese

Directions:

1. Whip the eggs and cream cheese in a bowl using a hand mixer on low speed.
2. Add the garlic, chives, sea salt, Italian seasoning, and mix into the egg cheese mixture.
3. Add the water, almond flour, heavy cream, and cheddar cheese. Mix well.
4. Slowly mix the sausage into the mixture using a spatula.

5. However, take a look at the manufacturer's instructions for mixing dry and wet ingredients.
6. Select the dough cycle setting, or specific muffin program, if available.
7. Then press start once you have closed the lid of the machine.
8. Remove dough from bread machine when the cycle is complete.
9. Grease a muffin pan with cooking spray.
10. Drop a heap mold of dough into 8 wells on the muffin top pan.
11. Bake in the oven for 25 minutes.
12. Cool and serve.

Nutrition:

Calories 321,

Fat: 28 g,

Carb 3.5 g,

Protein 13 g.

14. Garlic Bread

Preparation Time: 2-hours

Cooking Time: 40 – 50 Minutes

Servings: 8 Slices

Ingredients:

- 2 cups (8 ounces) almond flour
- 1 tsp. sea salt
- 1 Tbsp. keto baking powder
- 1 tsp. garlic powder
- 1 whole egg, beaten
- ½ cup (2 ounces) mozzarella cheese, shredded

For the Topping

- 1 tbsp. Unsalted butter, melted
- ¼ tbsp. Garlic powder
- ¼ tbsp. Sea salt
- ¾ cup (3 ounces) mozzarella cheese, shredded
- ½ tbsp. rosemary

Directions:

1. Prepare all of the ingredients for your bread and gather your measuring tools (a cup, a spoon, kitchen scales).
2. Close the cover.
3. Set your bread machine program to CAKE for 30 minutes (depending on the bread machine model) and choose the crust color LIGHT.
4. Press START.
5. Help the bread machine knead the dough with a spatula, if necessary.
6. After 10 minutes of baking, start checking for doneness using a toothpick. The approximate baking time is 10 - 15 minutes.
7. Using the garlic butter, brush the top of the bread, and then sprinkle with the shredded mozzarella cheese and rosemary.
8. When done, take the bucket out and let it cool for 5-10 minutes.
9. Shake the loaf from the pan and let cool for 20 minutes on a cooling rack.
10. Slice, serve and enjoy the taste of fragrant keto garlic bread.

Nutrition:

Calories 176;

Net Carbs 3.7g,

Total Fat 14.9g;

Saturated Fat 1.4g;

Cholesterol 21g;

Sodium 546mg;

Total Carbohydrate 6.7g;

Dietary Fiber 3g;

Total Sugars 1.1g;

Protein 7.3g,

Vitamin D 2mcg,

Calcium 95mg,

Iron 1mg,

Potassium 11mg

15. Feta Oregano Bread

Preparation Time: 1-hour

Cooking Time: 25 Minutes

Servings: 8

Ingredients:

- Almond flour, one cup
- Crumbled feta cheese, one cup
- Half cup of warm water
- Oregano dried, one teaspoon
- Baking powder, two-thirds of a teaspoon
- Extra virgin olive oil, a teaspoon
- Salt, half a teaspoon
- Swerve sweetener, one teaspoon
- Garlic powder, a quarter teaspoon
- Dried active yeast, one teaspoon

Directions:

1. In a mixing container, combine the almond flour, Swerve sweetener, dried oregano, baking powder, ground garlic, and salt.
2. In another mixing container, combine the extra virgin olive oil and warm water.
3. As per the instructions on your machine's manual, pour the ingredients in the bread pan, taking care to follow how to mix in the yeast.
4. Select the sweet bread setting, together with the bread size and crust type, if available, then press start once you have closed the machine's lid.
5. When the bread is ready, using oven mitts, remove the bread pan from the machine. Use a stainless spatula to extract the bread from the pan and turn the pan upside down on a metallic rack where the bread will cool off before slicing it.

Nutrition:

Calories: 166 calories

Total Carbohydrate: 26 g

Total Fat: 4g

Protein: 6 g

Sodium: 209 mg

16. Bacon Bread

Preparation Time: 2-hours

Cooking Time: 1 – 1½ Hours

Servings: 12 Slices

Ingredients:

- 7 oz. bacon, diced and fried
- 1/3 cup sour cream, room temperature

- 2 whole eggs, room temperature
- 4 Tbsp. salted butter, melted
- 1½ cup almond flour
- 1 Tbsp. keto baking powder
- 1 cup parmesan, grated

Directions:

1. Prepare all of the ingredients for your bread and gather your measuring tools (a cup, a spoon, kitchen scales).
2. Carefully whisk sour cream with eggs.
3. Mix all the ingredients into the bread machine pan and close the cover.
4. Set your bread machine program to cake for 45 – 60 minutes (depending on the bread machine model) and choose the crust color light.
5. Press start.
6. Help the bread machine knead the dough with a spatula, if necessary.
7. Before baking, sprinkle the top with grated cheese.
8. After 35 minutes of baking, start checking for doneness using a toothpick. The approximate baking time is 40 - 50 minutes.
9. Wait until the program is complete.
10. When done, take the bucket out and let it cool for 5-10 minutes.
11. Shake the loaf from the pan and let cool for 30 minutes on a cooling rack.
12. Slice, serve with a piece of butter and enjoy the taste of fragrant keto cheese bread.

Nutrition:

Calories 256;

Net Carbs 2.6g,

Total Fat 21.6g;

Saturated Fat 7,4g;

Cholesterol 63g;

Sodium 731mg;

Total Carbohydrate 4.1g;

Dietary Fiber 1.5g;

Total Sugars 0.6g;

Protein 12.8g,

Vitamin D 5mcg,

Calcium 148mg,

Iron 1mg,

Potassium 120mg

17. Mozzarella Herbs Bread

Preparation Time: 1-hour

Cooking Time: 15 Minutes

Servings: 10

Ingredients:
- 1 cup grated cheese mozzarella
- ½ cup grated cheese parmesan
- ½ teaspoon salt
- 1 teaspoon baking powder
- 1 cup almond flour
- 1 cup coconut flour
- ½ cup of warm water
- 1 teaspoon stevia
- ¼ teaspoon dried thyme
- 1 teaspoon grounded garlic

- 1 teaspoon dried basil
- 1 teaspoon olive oil extra virgin
- 2 teaspoons unsalted melted butter
- 1/3 cup unsweetened almond milk

Directions:

1. In a mixing container, mix the almond flour, baking powder, salt, parmesan cheese, mozzarella cheese, coconut flour, dried basil, dried thyme, garlic powder, and stevia powder.
2. Get another mixing container and mix warm water, unsweetened almond milk, melted unsalted butter, and extra virgin olive oil.
3. Select the basic bread setting, together with the bread size and crust type, if available, then press start once you have closed the machine's lid.
4. When the bread is ready, using oven mitts, remove the pan's bread from the machine. Use a stainless spatula to extract the bread from the pan and turn the pan upside down on a metallic rack where the bread will cool off before slicing it.

Nutrition:

Calories 49,

Fat 2 g,

Carb 2 g,

Protein 1 g

18. Cheesy Low Carb Butter & Garlic Bread

Preparation Time: 1-hour

Cooking Time: 15 Minutes

Servings: 16

Ingredients:

- For Bread:
- 4 tablespoons melted butter
- 5 eggs
- 2 tablespoons ricotta cheese
- 1 cup mozzarella cheese
- 1 cup cheddar cheese
- 1/3 cup parmesan cheese
- 2 cups almond flour
- 1/2 teaspoon xanthan gum
- 1 teaspoon Italian seasoning
- 1 teaspoon garlic powder
- 1 teaspoon oregano
- 1 teaspoon parsley
- 1 teaspoon salt
- For garlic butter spread
- 1 teaspoon garlic powder
- 2 tablespoons melted butter

Directions:

1. Prepare bread machine loaf pan greasing it with cooking spray.
2. In a bowl, mix dries ingredients until well combined.
3. Following the instructions on your machine's manual, mix the dry ingredients into the wet ingredients and pour in the bread machine loaf pan, taking care to follow how to mix in the baking powder.
4. Select the basic bread setting, together with the bread size and crust type, if available, then press start once you have closed the machine's lid.
5. When the bread is ready, using oven mitts, remove the bread pan from the machine.
6. Let it cool before slicing.

7. Whisk together melted butter and garlic in a small bowl until well blended. Brush with garlic butter and serve.

Nutrition:

Calories 240,

Total Fat 14 g,

Carb 4 g,

Dietary Fiber 1.5 g,

Sugars 1 g,

Protein 7 g,

Cholesterol 286 mg,

Sodium 302 mg

19.   Low-carb Bagel

Preparation Time: 2-hours

Cooking Time: 25 Minutes

Servings: 12

Ingredients:
- For Bagel:
- 1 cup Protein powder, unflavored
- 1/3 cup coconut flour
- 1 tsp. Baking powder
- ½ tsp. Sea salt
- ¼ cup ground flaxseed
- 1/3 cup sour cream
- 12 eggs

- Seasoning topping:
- 1 tsp. Dried parsley
- 1 tsp. Dried oregano
- 1 tsp. Dried minced onion
- ½ tsp. Garlic powder
- ½ tsp. Dried basil
- ½ tsp. Sea salt

Directions:

1. In a mixer, blend sour cream and eggs until well combined.
2. Whisk together the flaxseed, salt, baking powder, Protein powder, and coconut flour in a bowl.
3. Whisk the topping seasoning together in a small bowl. Set aside.
4. Following the instructions on your machine's manual, mix the dry ingredients into the wet ingredients and pour in the bread pan, following how to mix in the baking powder.
5. Select the basic bread setting, together with the bread size and crust type, if available, then press start once you have closed the machine's lid.
6. When the bread is ready, using oven mitts, remove the bread pan from the machine.
7. Sprinkle pan with about 1 tbsp. topping seasoning and evenly pour batter into each.
8. Sprinkle the top of each bagel evenly with the rest of the seasoning mixture.
9. Serve.

Nutrition:

Calories 134,

Fat 6.8 g,

Carb 4.2 g,

Protein 12.1 g

20. Cheese & Fruit Stuffed Panini

Preparation Time: 1-hour

Cooking Time: 30 Minutes

Servings: 10

Ingredients:

- Low carb flatbread (10 slices)
- 2 tbsp. Dijon mustard
- 2 tbsp. Mayonnaise
- 250g aged ham
- 120g brie thinly sliced
- 1 green apple very thinly sliced
- Oil or melted butter for brushing

Directions:

Chapter 1. Start by preheating your Panini maker.

Chapter 2. Cut through the center of each slice of bread to get two very flat and thin pieces.

Chapter 3. Spread one side of all the elements with the combined mustard and mayonnaise.

Chapter 4. Form sandwiches with the cheese and ham.

Chapter 5. Brush the sandwiches' outer parts with the melted butter and put in the Panini markers, leaving it grill until golden.

Nutrition:

Calories 288,

Total Fat 12 g,

Carb 15.5 g,

Dietary Fiber 7.1 g,

Protein 13.6 g,

Cholesterol 217 mg,

Sodium 329 mg

Chapter 7. Vegetable Breads

21. Beetroot Bread

Preparation Time: 1-hour

Cooking time: 2 hours

Servings: 10

Ingredients:

- 16 slice bread (1½ pounds)
- 1 cup lukewarm water
- 1 cup grated raw beetroot
- 2 tablespoons unsalted butter, melted
- 2 tablespoons sugar
- 2 teaspoons table salt
- 4 cups white bread flour
- 1⅔ teaspoons bread machine yeast

Directions:

1. Preparing the Ingredients.
2. Choose the size of the loaf of your preference and then measure the ingredients.
3. Add all of the ingredients mentioned previously in the list.
4. Close the lid after placing the pan in the bread machine.
5. Select the Bake cycle
6. Turn on the bread machine. Select the White/Basic setting; select the loaf size, and the crust color. Press start.

7. When the cycle is processed, remove the pan from the bread maker and let it rest.

8. Remove the bread from the pan; put it in a wire rack to cool for about 5 minutes. Slice

Nutrition:

Calories 288,

Total Fat 12 g,

Carb 15.5 g,

Dietary Fiber 7.1 g,

Protein 13.6 g,

22. Yeasted Carrot Bread

Preparation Time: 1-hour

Cooking time: 3 hours

Servings: 10

Ingredients:

- 12 slice bread
- ¾ cup milk
- 3 tablespoons melted butter, cooled
- 1 tablespoon honey
- 1½ cups shredded carrot
- ¾ teaspoon ground nutmeg
- ½ teaspoon salt

- 3 cups flour
- 2¼ teaspoons active dry yeast

Directions:

1. Preparing the Ingredients.
2. Choose the size of the loaf of your preference and then measure the ingredients.
3. Add all of the ingredients mentioned previously in the list.
4. Close the lid after placing the pan in the bread machine.
5. Select the Bake cycle
6. Turn on the bread machine. Select the Quick/Rapid setting, select the loaf size, and the crust color. Press start.
7. When the cycle is processed, remove the pan from the bread maker and let it rest.

Nutrition:

Calories 288,

Total Fat 12 g,

Carb 15.5 g,

Dietary Fiber 7.1 g,

Protein 13.6 g,

Cholesterol 217 mg,

Sodium 329 mg

23.   Basil Tomato Bread

Preparation Time: 1-hour

Cooking Time: 15 Minutes

Servings: 10

Ingredients:

- 12 slice bread (1½ pounds)
- ¾ cup lukewarm tomato sauce
- ¾ tablespoon olive oil
- ¾ tablespoon sugar
- ¾ teaspoon table salt
- 2¼ cups white bread flour
- 1½ tablespoons dried basil
- ¾ tablespoon dried oregano
- 3 tablespoons grated Parmesan cheese
- 2 teaspoons bread machine yeast

Directions:

1. Choose the size of a loaf of your preference and then measure the ingredients.
2. Add all of the ingredients mentioned previously in the list.
3. Close the lid after placing the pan in the bread machine.
4. Select the Bake cycle
5. Turn on the bread machine. Select the White/Basic setting; select the loaf size, and the crust color. Press start.

6. When the cycle is processed, remove the pan from the bread maker and let it rest.

7. Remove the bread from the pan; put it in a wire rack to cool for about 5 minutes. Slice

Nutrition:

Calories 134,

Fat 6.8 g,

Carb 4.2 g,

Protein 12.1 g

24. Savory Onion Bread

Preparation Time: 1-hour

Cooking time: 3 hours

Servings: 1 loaf

Ingredients:

- 12 slice bread (1½ pounds)
- 1 cup water, at 80°F to 90°F
- 3 tablespoons melted butter, cooled
- 1½ tablespoons sugar
- 1⅛ teaspoons salt
- 3 tablespoons dried minced onion
- 1½ tablespoons chopped fresh chives
- 3 tablespoons white bread flour

- 1⅔ teaspoons bread machine or instant yeast

Directions:

1. Preparing the Ingredients.
2. Group the ingredients in your bread machine.
3. Select the Bake cycle
4. Turn on the bread machine. Select the White/Basic setting, select the loaf size, and the crust color. Press start.
5. When the cycle is processed, remove the pan from the bread maker and let it rest.

Nutrition:

Calories 288,

Total Fat 12 g,

Carb 15.5 g,

Dietary Fiber 7.1 g,

Protein 13.6 g,

25. Confetti Bread

Preparation Time: 1-hour

Cooking time: 3 hours

Servings: 1 loaf

Ingredients:

- 8 slice bread
- ⅓ cup milk

- 2 cups of water
- 2 teaspoons melted butter, cooled
- ⅔ teaspoon white vinegar
- 4 teaspoons sugar
- ⅔ teaspoon salt
- 4 teaspoons grated Parmesan cheese
- ⅓ cup quick oats
- 1⅔ cups white bread flour
- 1 teaspoon bread machine or instant yeast
- ⅓ cup finely chopped zucchini
- ¼ cup finely chopped yellow bell pepper
- ¼ cup finely chopped red bell pepper
- 4 teaspoons chopped chives

Directions:

1. Preparing the Ingredients.
2. Place the ingredients, except the vegetables, in your bread machine as recommended by the manufacturer.
3. Select the Bake cycle
4. Set the machine for White bread, select light or medium crust, and press Start.
5. When the machine signals, add the chopped vegetables; if your machine has no signal, add the vegetables just before the second kneading is finished.
6. When the cycle is processed, remove the pan from the bread maker and let it rest.

Nutrition:

Calories 240,

Total Fat 14 g,

Carb 4 g,

Dietary Fiber 1.5 g,

Sugars 1 g,

Protein 7 g,

Cholesterol 286 mg,

26. Honey Potato Flakes Bread

Preparation Time: 10 minutes

Cooking time: 3 hours

Servings: 1 loaf

Ingredients:

- 12 slice bread (1½ pounds)
- 1¼ cups lukewarm milk
- 2 tablespoons unsalted butter, melted
- 1 tablespoon honey
- 1½ teaspoons table salt
- 3 cups white bread flour
- 1 teaspoon dried thyme
- ½ cup instant potato flakes
- 2 teaspoons bread machine yeast

Directions:

1. Preparing the Ingredients.
2. Choose the size of a loaf of your preference and then measure the ingredients.
3. Add all of the ingredients mentioned previously in the list.
4. Close the lid after placing the pan in the bread machine.
5. Select the Bake cycle
6. Turn on the bread machine. Select the White/Basic setting; select the loaf size, and the crust color. Press start.
7. When the cycle is processed, remove the pan from the bread maker and let it rest.

Nutrition:

Calories 162,

Fat 6 g,

Fiber 2 g,

Carbs 6 g,

Protein 4 g

27. Pretty Borscht Bread

Preparation Time: 10 minutes

Cooking time: 2 hours

Servings: 1 loaf

Ingredients:

- 12 slice bread

- ¾ cups water
- 1 ¾ cup grated raw beetroot
- 1½ tablespoons melted butter, cooled
- 1½ tablespoons sugar
- 1¼ teaspoons salt
- 3 cups white bread flour
- 1¼ teaspoons bread machine or instant yeast

Directions:

1. Preparing the Ingredients.
2. Group the ingredients in your bread machine.
3. Set the machine for Basic/White bread, select light or medium crust, and press Start.
4. Select the Bake cycle
5. When the loaf is processed, gently remove the bucket from the machine.
6. Shake the bucket to remove the loaf before slicing.

Nutrition:

Calories 200,

Fat 8 g,

Fiber 3 g,

Carbs 5 g,

Protein 6 g

28. Hot Red Pepper Bread

Preparation Time: 10 minutes

Cooking time: 2 hours

Servings: 1 loaf

Ingredients:

- 12 slice bread (1½ pounds)
- 1¼ cups milk, at 80°F to 90°F
- ¼ cup red pepper relish
- 2 tablespoons chopped roasted red pepper
- 3 tablespoons melted butter, cooled
- 3 tablespoons light brown sugar
- 1 teaspoon salt
- 3 cups white bread flour
- 1½ teaspoons bread machine or instant yeast

Directions:

1. Preparing the Ingredients.
2. Choose the size of the loaf of your preference and then measure the ingredients.
3. Add all of the ingredients mentioned previously in the list.
4. Close the lid after placing the pan in the bread machine.
5. Select the Bake cycle
6. Turn on the bread machine. Select the White/Basic setting; select the loaf size and the crust color. Press start.

7. When the cycle is processed, remove the pan from the bread maker and let it rest.

8. Remove the bread from the pan put it in a wire rack to cool for about 10 minutes. Slice

Nutrition:

Calories 106

Carbs: 21 g.

Fat: 1g.

Protein 2.8g

29. French Onion Bread

Preparation Time: 10 minutes

Cooking time: 2 hours

Servings: 1 loaf

Ingredients:

- 12 slice bread
- 1¼ cups milk
- 1 ¼ cup melted butter, cooled
- 3 tablespoons light brown sugar
- 1 teaspoon salt
- 3 tablespoons dehydrated onion flakes
- 2 tablespoons chopped fresh chives
- 1 teaspoon garlic powder

- 3 cups white bread flour
- 1 teaspoon bread machine or instant yeast

Directions:

1. Preparing the Ingredients.
2. Choose the size of the loaf of your preference and then measure the ingredients.
3. Add all of the ingredients mentioned previously in the list.
4. Close the lid after placing the pan in the bread machine.
5. Select the Bake cycle
6. Turn on the bread machine. Select the White/Basic setting; select the loaf size and the crust color. Press start.
7. When the cycle is processed, remove the pan from the bread maker and let it rest.
8. Remove the bread from the pan; put it in a wire rack to cool for about 5 minutes. Slice

Nutrition:

Calories 162,

Fat 6 g,

Fiber 2 g,

Carbs 6 g,

Protein 4 g

30. Garlic Onion Pepper Bread
Preparation Time: 1-Hour

Cooking time: 2 hours

Servings: 10

Ingredients:

- ½ cups of Water
- ¼ cup. chopped Onion
- ¼ cup. chopped Bell pepper
- 2 tsp. Chopped Garlic
- 2 tsp. butter
- 2 cups of bread flour
- 1 tbsp. Sugar
- 1 tsp. Cajun seasoning
- ½ tsp. Salt
- 1 tsp. Active dry yeast

Directions:

1. Take all ingredients into the bread machine pan. Select basic bread setting, then select medium crust and press start.
2. Once the loaf is done, remove the loaf pan from the machine. Allow it to cool for 10 minutes.
3. Slice and serve.

Nutrition:

Calories 106

Carbs: 21 g.

Fat: 1g.

Protein 2.8g

31. Healthy Banana Bread

Preparation Time: 1-hour

Cooking time: 2 hours

Servings: 10

Ingredients:

- 2 Eggs
- 1/3 cup. Butter
- 1/8 cup. Milk
- 2, mashed Bananas
- 1 1/3 cups of bread flour
- 2/3 cups of Sugar
- 1 ¼ tablespoon of Baking powder
- ½ tsp. Baking soda
- ½ tsp. Salt
- ½ cup. chopped Walnuts

Directions:

1. Add eggs, butter, milk, and bananas into the bread machine pan.
2. Mix all the remaining ingredients and add to the bread pan.
3. Select quick bread setting, then select light crust and press start. Once the loaf is done, remove the loaf pan from the machine. Allow it to cool for 10 minutes.
4. Slice and serve.

Nutrition:

Calories 303

Carbs: 32g.

Fat: 16g.

Protein: 7g

32. Mushroom Leek Bread

Preparation Time: 1-hour

Cooking Time: 2 hours

Servings: 10

Ingredients:

- 2 tbsps. Butter
- 2 cups Sliced Mushrooms
- ¾ cup sliced leeks
- 1 ½ tsps. Dried thyme
- 1 1/3 cup. Water
- 1 ½ tsps. Salt
- 2 tbsps. Honey
- 1 ¼ cups. Whole wheat flour
- 3 cups. Bread flour
- 1 tsp. Yeast

Directions:

1. Heat butter into the saucepan over medium-high heat.
2. Add leeks, mushrooms, and thyme and sauté until tender.
3. Transfer mushroom leek mixture into the bread machine pan.
4. Add remaining ingredients into the bread machine pan. The select basic setting then selects medium crust and start.
5. Once the loaf is done, remove the loaf pan from the machine. Allow it to cool for 10 minutes.
6. Slice and serve.

Nutrition:

Calories 143

Carbs: 25.9g.

Fat: 2.5g.

Protein: 3.9g

33. Greek Olive Cheese Bread

Preparation Time: 1-hour

Cooking Time: 2 hours

Servings: 10

Ingredients:

- ¾ cup crumbled Feta cheese
- 1 cups of Milk
- 1 tbsp. Olive oil
- 1 tsp. Salt
- 3 cups of bread flour
- ½ cup Olives pitted and chopped
- 1 tbsp. Sugar
- 2 tsps. Active dry yeast

Directions:

1. Take all ingredients into the bread machine pan.
2. The select basic setting then selects medium crust and start.
3. Once the loaf is done, remove the loaf pan from the machine. Allow it to cool for 10 minutes.
4. Slice and serve.

Nutrition:

Calories 205

Carbs: 32.2g.

Fat: 5.4g.

Protein: 6.6g

35. Garden Vegetable Bread

Preparation Time: 15 minutes.

Cooking Time: 3-hour

Servings: 14 slices

Ingredients:

- ½ cup warm buttermilk (60°F to 70°F)
- 3 tbsp. water (70°F to 80°F)
- 1 tbsp. canola oil
- ⅔ cup of shredded zucchini
- ¼ cup chopped red sweet pepper
- 2 tbsp. chopped green onions
- 2 tbsp. grated parmesan cheese
- 2 tbsp. sugar
- 1 tbsp. Salt
- ½ tbsp. lemon-pepper seasoning
- ½ cup old-fashioned oats
- 2½ cup bread flour
- 1½ tbsp. Of active dry yeast

Directions:

1. Add each ingredient to the bread machine in the order and at the temperature recommended by your bread machine manufacturer. Close the lid; select the basic bread, medium crust setting on your bread machine, and press start.
2. When the bread machine has finished baking, remove the bread and put it on a cooling rack.

Nutrition:

Calories 162,

Fat 6 g,

Fiber 2 g,

Carbs 6 g,

Protein 4 g

36. Potato Bread

Preparation Time: 15 minutes.

Cooking Time: 3-hour & 30 minutes

Servings: 14 slices

Ingredients:

- ¾ cup milk
- ½ cup water
- 2 Tbsp. canola oil
- 1½ tsp. salt
- 3 cups bread flour
- ½ cup instant potato flakes
- 1 Tbsp. Sugar

- ¼ tsp. white pepper
- 2 tsp. active dry yeast

Directions:

1. Add each ingredient to the bread machine in the order and at the temperature recommended by your bread machine manufacturer.
2. Close the lid; select the basic bread, medium crust setting on your bread machine, and press start.
3. When the bread machine has finished baking, remove the bread and put it on a cooling rack.

Nutrition:

Calories 303

Carbs: 32g.

Fat: 16g.

Protein: 7g

37. Carrot Coriander Bread

Preparation Time: 15 minutes.

Cooking Time: 3-hour

Servings: 14 slices

Ingredients:

- 2-3 freshly grated carrots,
- 1⅛ cup lukewarm water
- 2 tbsp. sunflower oil
- 4 tsp. freshly chopped coriander
- 2½ cups unbleached white bread flour
- 2 tsp. ground coriander

- 1 tsp. salt
- 5 tsp. sugar
- 4 tsp. easy blend dried yeast

Directions:

1. Add each ingredient to the bread machine in the order and at the temperature recommended by your bread machine manufacturer.
2. Close the lid; select the basic bread, medium crust setting on your bread machine, and press start.
3. When the bread machine has finished baking, remove the bread and put it on a cooling rack.

Nutrition:

Calories: 162 g.

Fat 6 g,

Fiber 2 g,

Carbs 6 g,

Protein 4 g

38. Perfect Sweet Potato Bread

Preparation Time: 1-hour

Cooking time: 3 hours

Servings: 10

Ingredients:

- 1, mashed Sweet potato
- 2 tbsps. Milk powder

- 1 ½ tsps. Salt
- 1/3 cup of Brown sugar
- 2 tbsps., softened Butter
- ½ tsp. Cinnamon
- 4 cups. Bread flour
- 1 tsp. Vanilla extract
- ½ cups of Warm water

Directions:

1. Add water, vanilla, bread flour, cinnamon, butter, brown sugar, salt, yeast, milk powder, and sweet potato into the bread machine pan.
2. Select white bread setting, then select light crust and press start.
3. Once the loaf is done, remove the loaf pan from the machine. Allow it to cool for 10 minutes.
4. Slice and serve.

Nutrition:

Calories 256

Carbs: 50.1g.

Fat: 2.9g.

Protein: 6.6g

39. **Potato Dill Bread**

Preparation Time: 15minutes.

Cooking Time: 40 minutes

Servings: 14 slices

Ingredients:

- 25-ounce package active dry yeast
- ½ cup water
- 1 tbsp. sugar
- 1 tbsp. salt
- 2 tbsp. melted butter
- 1 package or bunch fresh dill
- ¾ cup room temperature mashed potatoes
- 2¼ cups bread flour

Directions:

1. Add each ingredient to the bread machine in the order and at the temperature recommended by your bread machine manufacturer.
2. Close the lid; select the basic bread, medium crust setting on your bread machine, and press start.
3. When the bread machine has finished baking, remove the bread and put it on a cooling rack.

Nutrition:

Calories 100,

Fat: 6 g.

Carb 3 g,

Protein 11 g

40. Healthy Celery Loaf

Preparation Time: 2 hours 40 minutes

Cooking Time: 50 minutes

Servings: 1 loaf

Ingredients:

- 1 can cream of celery soup
- 3 tablespoons low-fat milk, heated
- 1 tablespoon vegetable oil
- 1¼ teaspoons celery salt
- ¾ cup celery, fresh/sliced thin
- 1 tablespoon celery leaves, fresh, chopped
- 1 whole egg
- ¼ teaspoon sugar
- 3 cups bread flour
- ¼ teaspoon ginger
- ½ cup quick-cooking oats
- 2 tablespoons gluten
- 2 teaspoons celery seeds
- 1 pack of active dry yeast

Directions:

1. Take all of the ingredients to your bread machine, carefully following the instructions of the manufacturer
2. Set the program of your bread machine to Basic/White Bread and set crust type to Medium
3. Press START
4. Wait until the cycle completes
5. Once the loaf is ready, take the bucket out and gently shake the bucket to remove the loaf
6. Slice, and serve

Nutrition:

Calories: 73 Cal

Fat: 4 g

Carbohydrates: 8 g

Protein: 3 g

Fiber: 1 g

Chapter 8. Gluten Free Bread

41. Gluten-Free Potato Bread

Preparation Time: 5 minutes

Cooking Time: 3 hours

Servings: 12

Ingredients:

- 1 medium russet potato, baked, or mashed leftovers
- 2 packets gluten-free quick yeast
- 3 tablespoons honey
- 3/4 cup warm almond milk
- 2 eggs, 1 egg white
- 3 2/3 cups almond flour
- 3/4 cup tapioca flour
- 1 teaspoon of sea salt
- 1 teaspoon dried chives
- 1 tablespoon apple cider vinegar
- 1/4 cup olive oil

Directions:

1. In a large bowl, mix all together with the ingredients, except for the yeast.
2. Whisk together the milk, eggs, oil, apple cider, and honey in a separate mixing bowl.
3. Pour the wet ingredients into the bread maker.
4. Group the dry ingredients over the wet ingredients.
5. Set to Gluten-Free bread setting, light crust color, and press Start.
6. Allow cooling completely before slicing.

Nutrition:

Calories: 232

Sodium: 173 mg

Dietary Fiber: 6.3 g.

Fat: 13.2 g.

Carbs: 17.4 g.

Protein: 10.4 g

42. Sorghum Bread Recipe

Preparation Time: 5 minutes

Cooking Time: 3 hours

Servings: 12

Ingredients:

- 1 cups sorghum flour
- 1 cup of tapioca starch
- 1/4cup brown or white sweet rice flour
- 1 ½ teaspoon xanthan gum
- 1 teaspoon guar gum
- 1/4 teaspoon salt
- 2 tablespoons sugar
- 2 teaspoons instant yeast
- 4 eggs (room temperature, lightly beaten)
- 1/2 cup oil
- 1 1/4 teaspoons vinegar
- 3/4-1 cup milk (105 - 115°F)

Directions:

1. Mix the ingredients, except for the yeast.
2. Set to Basic bread cycle, light crust color, and press Start.

3. Remove and lay on its side to cool on a wire rack before serving.

Nutrition:

Calories: 169

Sodium: 151 mg.

Dietary Fiber: 2.5 g.

Fat: 6.3 g.

Carbs: 25.8 g.

Protein: 3.3 g.

43. Gluten-Free Simple Sandwich Bread

Preparation Time: 5 minutes

Cooking Time: 1 hour

Servings: 12

Ingredients:

- 1 1/2 cups of sorghum flour
- 1 cup tapioca starch or potato starch
- ¼ cup gluten-free oat flour
- 2 teaspoons xanthan gum
- 1 1/4 teaspoons acceptable sea salt
- 2 1/2 teaspoons gluten-free yeast for bread machines
- 1 1/4 cups warm water
- 3 tablespoons extra virgin olive oil
- 1 tablespoon honey or raw agave nectar
- 1/2 teaspoon mild rice vinegar or lemon juice
- 2 organic free-range eggs, beaten

Directions:

1. In a large bowl, mix all together with the ingredients, except for the yeast.
2. Add the liquid ingredients to the bread maker pan first, and then gently pour the mixed dry ingredients on top of the liquid.
3. Set for Rapid 1 hour 20 minutes, medium crust color, and press Start.
4. Slice and ready to serve.

Nutrition:

Calories: 137

Sodium: 85 mg.

Dietary Fiber: 2.7 g.

Fat: 4.6 g.

Carbs: 22.1 g.

Protein: 2.4 g.

44. Gluten-Free Oat & Honey Bread

Preparation Time: 5 minutes

Cooking Time: 3 hours

Servings: 12

Ingredients:

- 1 1/4 cups warm water
- 3 tablespoons honey
- 2 eggs
- 3 tablespoons butter, melted
- 1 1/4 cups gluten-free oats
- 1 1/4 cups brown rice flour

- 1/2 cup potato starch
- 2 teaspoons xanthan gum
- 1 1/2 teaspoons sugar
- 3/4 teaspoon salt
- 1 1/2 tablespoons active dry yeast

Directions:

1. Add ingredients in the order listed above, except for the yeast.
2. Make a well in the center of the dry ingredients and add the yeast.
3. Select the Gluten-Free cycle, light crust color, and press Start.
4. Remove bread and allow the bread to cool on its side on a cooling rack for 20 minutes before slicing to serve.

Nutrition:

Calories: 151

Sodium: 265 mg.

Dietary Fiber: 4.3 g.

Fat: 4.5 g.

Carbs: 27.2 g.

Protein: 3.5 g.

45. Gluten-Free Cinnamon Raisin Bread

Preparation Time: 5 minutes

Cooking Time: 3 hours

Servings: 12

Ingredients:

- 3/4 cup almond milk

- 2 tablespoons flax meal
- 6 tablespoons warm water
- 1 1/2 teaspoons apple cider vinegar
- 2 tablespoons butter
- 1 1/2 tablespoons honey
- 1 2/3 cups brown rice flour
- 1/4 cup corn starch
- 2 tablespoons potato starch
- 1 1/2 teaspoons xanthan gum
- 1 tablespoon cinnamon
- 1/2 teaspoon salt
- 1 teaspoon active dry yeast
- 1/2 cup raisins

Directions:

1. Mix flax and water
2. Mix all the solid ingredients .except for the yeast.
3. Add wet ingredients to the bread machine.
4. Add the dry mixture on top and make a well in the middle of the dry.
5. Add the yeast to the well.
6. Set to Gluten-Free, light crust color, and press Start.
7. After the first kneading and rise cycle, add raisins.
8. Remove to a cooling rack when baked and let cool for 15 minutes before slicing.

Nutrition:

Calories: 192

Sodium: 173 mg.

Dietary Fiber: 4.4 g.

Fat: 4.7 g.

Carbs: 38.2 g.

Protein: 2.7 g.

46. Grain-Free Chia Bread

Preparation Time: 5 minutes

Cooking Time: 3 hours

Servings: 12

Ingredients:

- 1 cup warm water
- 3 large organic eggs, room temperature
- 1/4 cup olive oil
- 1 tablespoon apple cider vinegar
- 1 cup gluten-free chia seeds, ground to flour
- 1 cup almond meal flour
- 1/2 cup potato starch
- 1/4 cup coconut flour
- 3/4 cup millet flour
- 1 tablespoon xanthan gum
- 1 1/2 teaspoons salt
- 2 tablespoons sugar
- 3 tablespoons nonfat dry milk
- 6 teaspoons instant yeast

Directions:

1. Group the wet ingredients together and add to the bread maker pan.
2. Whisk dry ingredients, except yeast, together and add on top of wet ingredients.
3. Select Whole Wheat cycle, light crust color, and press Start.
4. Allow to cool completely before serving.

Nutrition:

Calories: 375,

Sodium: 462 mg,

Dietary Fiber: 22.3 g,

Fat: 18.3 g, Carbs: 42 g,

Protein: 12.2 g.

47. Gluten-Free Pizza Crust

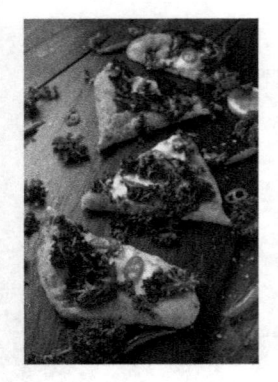

Preparation Time: 10 minutes

Cooking Time: 2 hours

Servings: 6 – 8

Ingredients:

- 3 large eggs, room temperature
- 1/2 cup olive oil
- 1 cup milk
- 1/2 cup water
- 2 cups of rice flour
- 1 cup cornstarch, and extra for dusting
- 1/2 cup potato starch
- 1/2 cup sugar
- 2 tablespoons yeast
- 3 teaspoons xanthan gum
- 1 teaspoon salt

Directions:

1. In a large bowl, mix all together with the ingredients, except for the yeast.
2. Combine the dry ingredients except for the yeast and add to the pan.
3. Select the Dough cycle and press Start.
4. When the dough is finished, press it out on a surface lightly sprinkled with corn starch and create a pizza shape. Use this dough with your favorite toppings and pizza recipe!

Nutrition:

Calories: 463

Sodium: 547 mg.

Dietary Fiber: 8.1 g.

Fat: 15.8 g.

Carbs: 79.2 g.

Protein: 7.4 g.

48. Gluten-Free Whole Grain Bread

Preparation Time: 15 minutes

Cooking Time: 3 hours 40 minutes

Servings: 12

Ingredients:

- 2/3 cup sorghum flour
- 1/2 cup buckwheat flour
- 1/2 cup millet flour
- 3/4 cup potato starch
- 2 1/4 teaspoons xanthan gum
- 1 1/4 teaspoons salt
- 3/4 cup skim milk
- 1/2 cup water
- 1 tablespoon instant yeast
- 5 teaspoons agave nectar, separated
- 1 large egg, lightly beaten
- 4 tablespoons extra virgin olive oil
- 1/2 teaspoon cider vinegar
- 1 tablespoon poppy seeds

Directions:

1. Whisk sorghum, buckwheat, millet, potato starch, xanthan gum, and sea salt in a bowl and set aside.
2. Combine milk and water in a glass measuring cup. Heat to between 110°F and 120°F; add 2 teaspoons of agave nectar and yeast and stir to combine.
3. Combine the egg, olive oil, remaining agave, and vinegar in another mixing bowl; add yeast and milk mixture. Pour wet ingredients into the bottom of your bread maker.
4. Top with dry ingredients.

5. Select the Gluten-Free cycle, light color crust, and press Start.
6. After the second kneading cycle, sprinkle with poppy seeds.
7. Remove pan from the bread to the machine. Enjoy!

Nutrition:

Calories: 153

Sodium: 346 mg.

Dietary Fiber: 4.1 g.

Fat: 5.9 g.

Carbs: 24.5 g.

Protein: 3.3 g

49. Gluten-Free Pull-Apart Rolls

Preparation Time: 5 minutes

Cooking Time: 2 hours

Servings: 9

Ingredients:

- 1 cup of warm water
- 2 tablespoons butter, unsalted
- 1 egg, room temperature
- 1 teaspoon apple cider vinegar
- 2 3/4 cups gluten-free almond-blend flour
- 1 1/2 teaspoons xanthan gum
- 1/4 cup sugar
- 1 teaspoon salt
- 2 teaspoons active dry yeast

Directions:

1. Add wet ingredients to the bread maker pan.
2. Mix dry ingredients except for yeast, and put in a pan.
3. Select the Dough cycle and press Start.
4. With non-stick cooking spray, spray an 8-inch round the cake pan
5. Roll the dough out into 9 balls, place a cake pan, and baste each with warm water.
6. Let rise for 1 hour.
7. Preheat oven to 400°F.
8. Bake for 30 minutes; until golden brown.
9. Brush with butter and serve.

Nutrition:

Calories: 568

Sodium: 380 mg.

Dietary Fiber: 5.5 g.

Fat: 10.5 g.

Carbs: 116.3 g.

Protein: 8.6 g.

50. Classic Gluten-Free Bread

Preparation Time: 5 minutes

Cooking Time: 15 minutes

Servings: 12

Ingredients:

- ½ cup butter, melted

- 3 tbsp. of coconut oil, melted
- 6 eggs
- 2/3 cup sesame seed flour
- 1/3 cup coconut flour
- 2 tsp. baking powder
- 1 tsp. psyllium husks
- ½ tsp. xanthan gum
- ½ tsp. salt

Directions:

1. Pour in eggs, melted butter, and melted coconut oil into your bread machine pan.
2. Add the remaining ingredients to the bread machine pan.
3. Set bread machine to gluten-free.
4. When the bread is cool, remove the bread machine pan from the bread machine.
5. You can store your bread for up to 3 days.

Nutrition:

Calories 146

Carbohydrates 1.2 g

Fats 14 g

Protein 3.5 g

51. Gluten-Free Chocolate Zucchini Bread

Preparation Time: 5 minutes

Cooking Time: 15 minutes

Servings: 12

Ingredients:

- 1 ½ cups coconut flour
- ¼ cup unsweetened cocoa powder
- ½ cup erythritol
- ½ tsp. cinnamon
- 1 tsp. baking soda
- 1 tsp. baking powder
- ¼ tsp. salt
- ¼ cup coconut oil, melted
- 4 eggs
- 1 tsp. vanilla
- 2 cups zucchini, shredded

Directions:

1. Shred the zucchini and use a tissue to drain excess water, set aside.
2. Lightly beat eggs with coconut oil, then add to bread machine pan.
3. Add the remaining ingredients to the pan.
4. Set bread machine to gluten-free.
5. When the bread is cool, remove the bread machine pan from the bread machine.
6. You can store your bread for up to 5 days.

Nutrition:

Calories 185

Carbohydrates 6 g

Fats 17 g

Protein 5 g

52. Honey Oat Bread

Preparation Time: 15 minutes

Cooking Time: 3 hours

Servings: 8

Ingredients:

- Dry Ingredients:
- 2 1/3 cups pure oat flour
- 1 cup pure rolled oats
- 2 ¼ teaspoons baking powder
- 1 ¼ teaspoons salt
- 1 teaspoon baking soda
- Wet Ingredients:
- 1 egg
- 1 cup yogurt, plain
- ¾ cup almond milk
- ¼ cup of coconut oil
- ¼ cup honey

Directions:

1. Add all wet ingredients first in the bread pan before the dry ingredients.
2. Press the "Basic" or "Normal" mode of the bread machine.
3. Select "Medium" as the crust color setting.
4. Wait until the device finishes the mixing, kneading, and baking cycles.
5. Take out the bread from the device.
6. Let it cool and serve.

Nutrition:

Calories: 181

Carbohydrates: 24g

Fat: 7g

Protein: 7g

53. Nutty Cinnamon Bread

Preparation Time: 10 minutes

Cooking Time: 2 hours

Servings: 8

Dry Ingredients:

- 3 ½ cups gluten-free self-rising flour
- ½ cup pecans, chopped
- ¼ cup butter
- 3 tablespoons brown sugar
- 1 ½ tablespoons powdered milk
- 2 teaspoons cinnamon
- 1 teaspoon salt

Wet Ingredients:

- 1 ¼ cups water

Directions:

1. Pour the water first into the bread pan, and then add the dry ingredients.
2. Select the "Normal" or "Basic" mode of the bread machine with the light crust color setting.
3. Allow the machine to complete all cycles.
4. Remove the bread from the machine.
5. Cool down completely before slicing the bread.

Nutrition:

Calories: 141

Carbohydrates: 21g

Fat: 25g

Protein: 3g

54. Nisus Bread

Preparation Time: 10 minutes

Cooking Time: 2 hours

Servings: 8

Dry Ingredients:

- 4 cups gluten-free self-rising flour
- ½ cup of sugar
- 3 tablespoons butter
- 1 teaspoon ground cardamom
- 1 teaspoon salt

Wet Ingredients:

- 1 egg
- 1 cup evaporated milk
- ¼ cup of water

Directions:

1. Add the wet ingredients first to the bread pan before adding the dry ingredients.
2. Press the "Normal" or "Basic" mode and light crust setting on the bread machine.
3. Wait until every cycle is through.
4. Cool down the bread completely.
5. Slice and serve.

Nutrition:

Calories: 184

Carbohydrates: 31g

Fat: 27g

Protein: 5g

55. Maple Syrup Spice Bread

Preparation Time: 15 minutes

Cooking Time: 3 hours

Servings: 10

Dry Ingredients:

- 2 ½ cups bread flour
- ½ cup raisins
- ¼ cup of sugar
- 1 tablespoon maple syrup
- 1 tablespoon cinnamon
- 1 tablespoon dried orange peel, minced
- 1 ½ teaspoons yeast
- ½ teaspoon nutmeg

Wet Ingredients:

- ¾ cup almond milk
- 3 tablespoons aquafaba
- 2 tablespoons vegetable oil

Directions:

1. Put all wet ingredients into the bread pan.

2. Add the dry ingredients.
3. Use the "Normal" or "Basic" mode and light crust color setting of your bread machine.
4. Wait until the cycles are over.
5. Move the bread to a wire rack.
6. Slice the bread and serve.

Nutrition:

Calories: 168

Carbohydrates: 30g

Fat: 3g

Protein: 4g

56. Cherry-Blueberry Loaf

Preparation Time: 10 minutes

Cooking Time: 3 hours

Servings: 1 loaf

Dry Ingredients:

- 4 cups bread flour
- ¼ cup brown sugar
- 1/3 cup dried cherries, chopped
- 1/3 cup dried blueberries, chopped
- 2 teaspoons yeast
- 1 ½ teaspoons salt

Wet Ingredients:

- 1 cup of water
- 2 tablespoons vegetable oil

Directions:

1. After pouring the water and oil into the bread pan, add the dry ingredients into the mix.
2. Press the "Normal" or "Basic" mode of the bread machine.
3. Choose either a light or medium crust color setting.
4. Once the cycles are done, transfer the bread to a wire rack.
5. Cool down the bread completely before slicing.

Nutrition:

Calories: 145

Carbohydrates: 29g

Fat: 2g

Protein: 4g

57. Gluten-Free Loaf

Preparation Time: 5 minutes

Cooking Time: 15 minutes

Servings: 12

Ingredients:

- ½ cup butter, melted
- 3 tbsp. coconut oil, melted
- 6 eggs
- 2/3 cup sesame seed flour
- 1/3 cup coconut flour
- 2 tsp. baking powder
- 1 tsp. psyllium husks
- ½ tsp. xanthan gum

- ½ tsp. salt

Directions:

1. Pour in eggs, melted butter, and melted coconut oil into your bread machine pan.
2. Add the remaining ingredients to the bread machine pan.
3. Set bread machine to gluten-free.
4. When the bread is done, remove the bread machine pan from the bread machine.
5. You can store your bread for up to 3 days.

Nutrition:

Calories 146

Carbohydrates 1.2 g

Fats 14 g

Protein 3.5 g

58. Healthy Grain-Free Bagels

Preparation Time: 10 minutes

Cooking time: 20 minutes

Servings: 6

Ingredients:

- 1/4 cup sour cream
- 1 1/2 cups almond flour
- 3 eggs

Directions:

1. Preheat your oven to 350 degrees. Grease five wells in a donut pan; set aside.

2. Beat eggs until creamy and light; stir in sour cream until very smooth. Mix in almond flour until well combined. Spread the batter into the donut molds; bake for about 20 minutes. Let cool and slice to serve. Best served toasted with sour cream or butter.

Nutrition:

Calories 270,

Fat 15,

Fiber 3,

Carbs 5,

Protein 9

59. Cream of Orange Bread

Preparation Time: 20 minutes

Cooking Time: 2.5 to 3 hours

Servings: 8

Dry Ingredients:

- 2 cups of rice flour
- ¾ cup potato flour
- ¼ cup tapioca flour
- 3 tablespoons sugar
- 2 tablespoons orange zest, minced
- 1 tablespoon xanthan gum
- 2 ¼ teaspoons active dry yeast
- 1 teaspoon lemon zest, minced
- 1 teaspoon salt
- ¼ teaspoon cardamom

Wet Ingredients:

- 3 eggs
- ¾ cup milk, half-and-half
- ¾ cup of water
- 3 tablespoons vegetable oil

Directions:

1. Add first the wet ingredients into the bread pan, then the dry ingredients.
2. Set the bread machine to "Basic," "Normal," or "White" mode.
3. Allow the machine to finish the mixing and baking cycles.
4. Take out the pan from the machine.
5. Wait for 10 minutes before transferring the bread to a wire rack.
6. When the bread has completely cooled down, slice it and serve.

Nutrition:

Calories: 190

Carbohydrates: 30g

Fat: 6g

Protein: 4g

60. Gluten-Free Crusty Boule Bread

Preparation Time: 15 minutes

Cooking Time: 3 hours

Servings: 12

Ingredients:

- 3 1/4 cups gluten-free flour mix
- 1 tablespoon active dry yeast

- 1 1/2 teaspoons kosher salt
- 1 tablespoon guar gum
- 1 1/3 cups warm water
- 2 large eggs, room temperature
- 2 tablespoons, plus 2 teaspoons olive oil
- 1 tablespoon honey

Directions:

1. Group all of the dry ingredients, in a large mixing bowl; set aside.
2. Group together the water, eggs, oil, and honey in a separate mixing bowl.
3. Pour the wet ingredients into the bread maker.
4. Add the dry ingredients over the wet ingredients.
5. Set to Gluten-Free setting and press Start.
6. Remove baked bread and allow cooling completely. Hollow out and fill with soup or dip to use as a boule or slice for serving.

Nutrition:

Calories 270,

Fat 15,

Fiber 3,

Carbs 5,

Protein 9

Chapter 9. Sourdough Breads

61. Sourdough Starter

Preparation Time: 5 days

Cooking Time:

Servings: 10

Ingredients:

- 2 cups of warm water
- 1 tablespoon sugar
- 1 active dry yeast
- 2 cups flour
- 1 proper container
- 1 spoon for stirring

Directions:

Day 1:

1. Mix the yeast, sugar, water, and whisk to combine. Exert the flour until well combined, and transfer to your container. Let it cover in a warm spot for 24 hours.

Day 2 - 4

1. Unlike the traditional starter, you don't need to feed this one yet. Stir it once or twice every 24 hours.

Day 5:

1. By now, the starter should have developed the classic slightly sour smell. If not, don't worry; you need to let it sit a bit longer. If it is ready, store it in the fridge, and feed it once a week until you're ready to use it. As with the traditional starter, you'll need to provide it the day before you plan to use it.

Nutrition:

Calories: 26 Cal

Fat: 0 g

Carbohydrates: 6 g

Protein: 1 g

62. Garlic And Herb Flatbread Sourdough

Preparation Time: 1 hour

Cooking Time: 25- 30 minutes

Servings: 12

Ingredients:

Dough

- 1 cup sourdough starter, fed or unfed
- 3/4 cup warm water
- 2 teaspoons instant yeast
- 3 cups all-purpose flour
- 1 1/2 teaspoons salt
- 3 tablespoons olive oil

Topping

- 1/2 teaspoon dried thyme
- 1/2 teaspoon dried oregano
- 1/2 teaspoon dried marjoram
- 1 teaspoon garlic powder
- 1/4 teaspoon onion powder
- 1/4 teaspoon salt

- 1/4 teaspoon pepper
- 3 tablespoons olive oil

Directions:

1. Take all the dough ingredients in the bowl of a stand mixer, and knead until smooth. Put in a lightly greased bowl and let rise for at least one hour. Punch down, and then let rise again for at least one hour.
2. To prepare the topping, mix all ingredients except the olive oil in a small bowl.
3. Lightly grease a standard baking sheet, and pat and roll the dough in the pan. Brush the olive oil over the dough, and sprinkle the herb and seasoning mixture over the top. Cover and let rise for 15-20 minutes.
4. Preheat oven to 420F and bake for 30 minutes.

Nutrition:

Calories: 89 Cal

Fat: 3.7 g

Protein: 1.8 g

63. Dinner Rolls

Preparation Time: 3 hours

Cooking Time: 5-10 minutes

Servings: 24 rolls

Ingredients:

- 1 cup sourdough starter
- 1 1/2 cups warm water
- 1 tablespoon yeast
- 1 tablespoon salt
- 2 tablespoons sugar

- 2 tablespoons olive oil
- 5 cups all-purpose flour
- 2 tablespoons butter, melted

Directions:

1. Mix the sourdough starter, water, yeast, salt, sugar, and oil. Add the flour. Take the dough in a greased bowl, and let it rise until doubled in size, about 2 hours.
2. Place the dough from a bowl on a table and divide it into 3-4 inch sized pieces. Place the buns into a greased 9x13 pan, and let them rise, covered, for about an hour.
3. Preheat the oven and bake the rolls for 15 minutes. Remove from the oven, brush with the melted butter, and bake for an additional 5-10 minutes.

Nutrition:

Calories: 128 Cal

Fat: 2.4 g

Protein: 3.2 g

Sugar: 1.1 g

64. Sourdough Boule

Preparation Time: 4 hours

Cooking Time: 25-35 minutes

Servings: 12

Ingredients:

- 275g Warm Water
- 500g sourdough starter
- 550g all-purpose flour
- 20g Salt

Directions:

1. Combine the flour, warm water, starter, and let sit, covered for at least 30 minutes.
2. After letting it sit, stir in the salt, and turn the dough out onto a floured surface. Flatten the dough slightly (it's best to "slap" it onto the counter), then fold it in half a few times.
3. Cover the dough and let it rise. Repeat the slap and fold a few more times. Now cover the dough and let it rise for 2-4 hours.
4. When the dough at least doubles in size, gently pull it, so the top of the dough is taught. Repeat several times. Let it rise for 2-4 hours once more.
5. Preheat to oven to 475F and either places a baking stone or a cast iron pan in the oven to preheat. Place the risen dough on the rock or pot, and score the top in several spots. Bake for 30 minutes

Nutrition:

Calories: 243 Cal

Fat: 0.7 g

Protein: 6.9 g

65. Herbed Baguette

Preparation Time: 45 minutes

Cooking Time: 20-25 minutes

Servings: 12

Ingredients:

- 1 1/4 cups warm water
- 2 cups sourdough starter, either fed or unfed
- 4 to 5 cups all-purpose flour

- 2 1/2 teaspoons salt
- 2 teaspoons sugar
- 1 tablespoon instant yeast
- 1 tablespoon fresh oregano, chopped
- 1 teaspoon fresh rosemary, chopped
- 1 tablespoon fresh basil, chopped

Directions:

1. Combine all ingredients, knead with a dough hook (or use your hands) until smooth dough forms -- about 7 to 10 minutes, if needed, add more flour.
2. Place the dough in an oiled bowl, cover, and allow rising for about 2 hours.
3. Divide the dough into 3 pieces. Shape each piece of dough for about 16 inches long. Do this by moving the dough into a log, folding it, rolling it into a log, then folding it and rolling it again.
4. Place the rolled baguette dough onto lined baking sheets, and cover. Let rise for one hour.
5. Preheat oven to 425F, and bake for 20-25 minutes

Nutrition:

Calories: 197 Cal

Fat: 0.6 g

Protein: 5.8 g

66. Pumpernickel Bread

Preparation Time: 2 hours 10 minutes

Cooking Time: 50 minutes

Servings: 1 loaf

Ingredients:

- 1 1/8 cups warm water
- 1 ½ tablespoon vegetable oil
- 1/3 cup molasses
- 3 tablespoons cocoa
- 1 tablespoon caraway seed (optional)
- 1 ½ teaspoon salt
- 1 ½ cups of bread flour
- 1 cup of rye flour
- 1 cup whole wheat flour
- 1 ½ tablespoon of vital wheat gluten (optional)
- 2 ½ teaspoon of bread machine yeast

Directions:

1. Mix them all and place them in the device.
2. Choose a basic bread cycle.
3. Take the bread out to cool and enjoy!

Nutrition:

Calories: 97 Cal

Fat: 1 g

Carbohydrates: 19 g

Protein: 3 g

67. Sauerkraut Rye

Preparation Time: 2 hours 20 minutes

Cooking Time: 50 minutes

Servings: 1 loaf

Ingredients:

- 1 cup sauerkraut, rinsed and drained
- ¾ cup of warm water
- 1½ tablespoons molasses
- 1½ tablespoons butter
- 1½ tablespoons brown sugar
- 1 teaspoon caraway seeds
- 1½ teaspoons salt
- 1 cup rye flour
- 2 cups bread flour
- 1½ teaspoons active dry yeast

Directions:

1. Mix all the ingredients.
2. Set the program of your bread machine to Basic/White Bread and set crust type to Medium
3. Press START
4. Wait until the cycle completes
5. Once the loaf is ready, take the bucket out.
6. To remove the loaf, gently shake the bucket
7. Slice, and serve

Nutrition:

Calories: 74 Cal

Fat: 2 g

Carbohydrates: 12 g

Protein: 2 g

Fiber: 1 g

68. Crusty Sourdough Bread

Preparation Time: 15 minutes; 1 week (Starter)

Cooking Time: 3 hours

Servings: 1 loaf

Ingredients:

- 1/2 cup water
- 3 cups bread flour
- 2 tablespoons sugar
- 1 ½ teaspoon of salt

Directions:

1. Measure 1 cup of starter and remaining bread ingredients, add to bread machine pan.
2. Choose basic/white bread cycle with medium or light crust color.

Nutrition:

Calories: 165 calories;

Total Carbohydrate: 37 g

Total Fat: 0 g

Protein: 5 g

Sodium: 300 mg

Fiber: 1 g

69. Honey Sourdough Bread

Preparation Time: 15 minutes; 1 week (Starter)

Cooking Time: 3 hours

Servings: 1 loaf

Ingredients:

- 2/3 cup sourdough starter
- 1/2 cup water
- 1 tablespoon vegetable oil
- 2 tablespoons honey
- 1/2 teaspoon salt
- 1/2 cup high protein wheat flour
- 2 cups bread flour
- 1 teaspoon active dry yeast

Directions:

1. Measure 1 cup of starter and remaining bread ingredients, add to bread machine pan.
2. Choose basic/white bread cycle with medium or light crust color.

Nutrition:

Calories: 175

Total Carbohydrate: 33 g

Total Fat: 0.3 g

Protein: 5.6 g

Sodium: 121 mg

Fiber: 1.9 g

70.   **Multigrain Sourdough Bread**

Preparation Time: 15 minutes: 1 week (Starter)

Cooking Time: 3 hours

Servings: 1 loaf

Ingredients:

- 2 cups starter sourdough
- 2 tablespoons butter
- 1/2 cup fresh milk
- ½ teaspoon salt
- 1/4 cup pure honey
- 1/4 cup sunflower seeds
- 1 1/2 cup millet or 1/2 cup amaranth or 1/2 cup quinoa
- 3 1/2 cups multi-grain flour

Directions:

1. Add ingredients to bread machine pan.
2. Choose the dough cycle.
3. Conventional Oven:
4. Shape the dough into a loaf.
5. Cover it, and rise until bread is a couple of inches above the edge.
6. Bake for 50 minutes.

Nutrition:

Calories: 110 calories;

Total Carbohydrate: 13.5 g

Total Fat: 1.8 g

Protein: 2.7 g

Sodium: 213 mg

Fiber: 1.4 g

71. Everyday Sourdough Bread

Preparation Time: 10 minutes

Cooking Time: 40-50 minutes

Servings: 18

Ingredients:

- 2 ½ cups All-purpose flour
- 2 cups sourdough starter
- 1 ½ tsp. Sugar Water, lukewarm
- 1 ½ tsp. Salt

Directions:

1. Group all the ingredients in a mixing bowl or the bowl of a stand mixer or food processor.
2. Place the dough inside. Set the bowl aside for 45-60 minutes for the dough to rise. The risen dough should be puffy but not necessarily have doubled in size.
3. Place the dough and gently punch the dough down to deflate.
4. Form the dough into a log of about 9 inches and place it into the prepared pan.
5. Cover the pan with a kitchen cloth or plastic wrap and allow the dough to rise for 60-90 minutes.
6. Switch on the oven 60 minutes into the second rising
7. Bake the bread until it has a light golden color, for 40-50 minutes. The bread is done when you insert a digital thermometer into the center, and it reads 190 degrees F (88 degrees C).
8. Remove the bread from the device and then place on a cooling rack to cool to room temperature before serving.

9. This bread can be stored well-wrapped for a number of days at room temperature. Nutrition

Nutrition:

Calories 110

Carbs 23 g

Fat 0 g

72. Cracked Wheat Bread

Preparation Time: 30 minutes

Cooking Time: 30 minutes

Servings: 12

Ingredients:

- ¼ cup Cracked wheat
- 1 cup Whole wheat flour
- 1 ¾ cups Bread flour
- 1 ¼ cup Sourdough starter
- ½ cup of Water, hot
- ¼ cup Flax seeds
- ¼ cup Sunflower seeds, raw
- 2 tbsp. Margarine, melted
- 1 tbsp. Molasses
- 1 tbsp. Honey
- ¼ cup nonfat milk

Directions:

1. Place the cracked wheat into a medium-sized bowl and pour the hot water over it. (Please note that the water does not need to be at the boiling point, just hot).
2. Add the flax seeds, melted margarine, nonfat milk, sunflower seeds, honey, and molasses and mix through.
3. Once the mixed ingredients have cooled to lukewarm, add the sourdough starter and stir.
4. Add the flours gradually 1 cup at a time. Start off with the whole wheat and then the bread flour, and use a sturdy wooden spoon to stir.
5. When the dough is stiff enough, turn it out onto a lightly floured work surface and knead for 10-12 minutes. Add some of the remaining flour if necessary, but it is not essential that you use all the flour.
6. Once the dough is elastic and smooth, use your hands to shape it into a ball.
7. Place the dough bowl and cover.
8. Leave the bowl in a draft-free place in the kitchen for 1 ½ hour until the dough has doubled in size.
9. Hit the dough down and again cover the dough with a kitchen cloth or plastic wrap. Allow the dough to rise for a second time for about 1 hour until it has again risen to double the size.
10. Punch the dough down again and shape the dough into an oblong log and place it into a greased loaf pan. Set the loaf pan aside for the dough to rise for the third time for 1 hour.
11. Make an egg wash of 1 tbsps. of water and 1 whole egg, whisked well
12. Switch the oven on about 30 minutes before the end of the third rising session and preheat to 375 degrees.

13. Bake the bread for about 30 minutes. After 15 minutes, spray the pan with cold water and continue baking.

14. Let the bread to cool down. Then place the loaf on the cooling rack to cool down completely before slicing.

Nutrition:

Calories 110

Carbs 23 g

Fat 0 g

Protein 4 g

73. Pumpkin Spice Sourdough Loaf

Preparation Time: 15 minutes

Cooking Time: 1 hour to 1 hour 30 minutes

Servings: 16

Ingredients:

- 2 cups All-purpose flour
- ¾ cup Sourdough starter unfed/discard
- ⅓ cup Vegetable oil
- ½ tsp. Ginger
- ½ cup Sugar
- ½ tsp. Cloves
- ¼ cup Molasses
- ¼ tsp. Nutmeg

- 2 Eggs, large
- ½ tsp. Baking powder
- 1 cup Pumpkin purée
- ½ tsp. Baking soda
- 1 tsp. Vanilla extract
- ½ cup Walnuts, chopped
- ¾ tsp. Salt
- ½ cup Raisins
- ½ tsp. Cinnamon

Directions:

1. Grease a loaf pan and set aside.
2. Place the sugar, pumpkin, oil, eggs, and molasses into a large mixing bowl and stir. Add the vanilla and the sourdough starter and stir again.
3. In a separate bowl, whisk the baking soda, flour, baking powder, salt, and spices together.
4. Add the dry ingredients to the bowl holding the wet ingredients and combine until all the ingredients are blended.
5. Stir the raisins and the nuts into the batter.
6. Pour the batter into the prepared loaf pan and place it into the oven.
7. Bake for 60-65 minutes and do a test for doneness by inserting a paring knife into the center of the loaf.
8. Remove from the device and place the loaf pan on a cooling rack, before turning the loaf out onto the cooling rack.
9. Let the pumpkin bread to cool completely and slice.

Nutrition:

Calories 110

Carbs 23 g

Fat 0 g

Protein 4 g

74. Sourdough Bread Sticks

Preparation Time: 25 minutes

Cooking Time: 20 to 30 minutes

Servings: 6

Ingredients:

- 2 cups all-purpose flour
- ½ cup Sourdough starter
- ½ tsp. Active dry yeast
- ½ cup   Water, warm
- ½ tbsps. sugar,
- ½ tsp.   Salt
- 1/2 Egg, separated

Directions:

1. Place half the sugar and water into a bowl and dissolve. Add yeast and set aside 5-10 minutes until the mixture is foamy.

2. Put the rest of the sugar, salt, and flour into a large mixing bowl and mix.

3. Put the egg yolk and sourdough starter in a separate bowl and combine. Put the egg white in a separate bowl and whisk and place it in the refrigerator until needed.

4. Add the sourdough and the yeast mixture to the dry ingredients. Use a wooden spoon and mix until all the ingredients are blended and the mixture holds together in soft dough.

5. Spray a large bowl with the vegetable oil and place the dough ball and cover, and let the dough rise.

6. Hit the dough down. Roll the dough balls into breadsticks of about 3-4 inches (7.6-10 cm) long. Place the breadsticks onto a baking sheet lined with parchment paper and cover with a cloth. Set aside to rest for 45 minutes.

7. Preheat the oven to 350 degrees.

8. Bake the breadsticks for 15-20 minutes until light brown. Bush the tops with egg white using a pastry brush. Bake it for 5-10 minutes until the breadsticks are medium brown.

9. Allow to cool down about 10 minutes before serving with toppings of your own choice.

Nutrition:

Calories 110

Carbs 23 g

Fat 0 g

Protein 4 g

75. Cheddar Sourdough Bread

Preparation Time: 45 minutes

Cooking Time: 60

Servings: 8

Ingredients:

- *3 cups bread flour + extra for dusting*
- ½ to 1 cup sour cream, based on dough's consistency
- 1 (17.6 ounces) unsweetened Greek yogurt
- 1 tsp. instant dry yeast
- 1 ¾ tsp. salt
- 4 ounces cheddar cheese, cut into ½-inch cubes

**Directions*:*

1. In a medium bowl, mix flour, sour cream, Greek yogurt, and yeast until sticky dough forms. Cover bowl with a plastic wrap and let sit at room temperature for 20 minutes.

2. After, remove plastic wrap and sprinkle salt on the dough. Gently knead salt into dough until well incorporated. Cover again with a plastic wrap and let rise at room temperature for 30 minutes. Remove wrap after.

3. Holding two edges of the dough with your fingertips, fold the dough over itself into the center. Turn bowl to a 45-degree angle, fold again and repeat this process six more times. Cover the dough. Repeat folding dough at 30 minute-intervals three more times.

4. Dust a clean, flat, working surface with flour. After the fourth and final fold, transfer dough to surface. Gently spread the dough into an 8-inch disk and then fold edges towards the center until round.

5. Press dough, add cheddar cheese cubes, and fold dough one more time into a round, making sure ingredients are well-incorporated; place seam-side on a

working surface. Loosely cup your hands and mold dough into a round shape while moving around. If the dough is too tacky, dust your hands with some flour and mold.

6. Line Benetton basket with its cover or clean napkin and dust with flour. Place dough in the basket, and cover lid. Wrap basket with a large plastic bag and tie tightly to cover basket fully. Let sit at room temperature, then refrigerate for 12 to 24 hours.

7. After, fix the oven's rack in the middle and sit a cake pan at the oven's bottom. Pour 3 cups of water into the cake pan and place the bannerol basket on the rack.

8. Remove basket and cake pan with water. Cut out a 12 x 12-inch greaseproof paper and spray with cooking spray. Unwrap basket, uncover lid, and dust top of the dough with flour.

9. Lay oiled side of the paper over the dough and inverted basket onto the counter; lift basket and cloth.

10. Pick up the dough while holding edges of parchment paper and lower into Dutch oven.

11. Heat oven to 425ºF and bake bread for 30 minutes once the oven is on. Uncover the pot and bake bread further for 20 to 30 minutes or until deep brown.

12. When ready, carefully remove the hot pot, transfer bread to a wire rack and let it completely cool for 2 hours.

13. Slice and enjoy bread afterward.

Nutrition:

Calories 110

Carbs 23 g

Fat 0 g

Protein 4 g

76. Spicy Cheddar Sourdough Bread

Preparation Time: 45 minutes

Cooking Time: 60 minutes

Servings: 8

Ingredients:

- *15 ½ ounces all-purpose flour + extra for dusting*
- 10 ounces water, room temperature
- 8 ounces sourdough starter
- 1 ¾ tsp. salt
- 1/3 cup sliced jalapeno peppers
- ¼ cup minced scallions
- 1 heaped cup grated cheddar cheese

Directions:

1. In a medium bowl, mix flour, water, and sourdough starter until sticky dough forms. Cover bowl with a plastic wrap and let sit at room temperature for 20 minutes.
2. After, remove plastic wrap and sprinkle salt on top; knead the dough until well incorporated. Cover again with a plastic wrap and let rise at room temperature for 30 minutes. Remove wrap after.
3. Holding two edges of the dough with your fingertips, fold the dough over itself into the center. Turn bowl to a 45-degree angle, fold again and repeat this

process six more times. Cover the dough and let rise. Repeat folding dough at 30 minute-intervals three more times.

4. Dust a clean, flat working surface with flour. After the fourth and final fold, transfer dough to the surface. Gently spread dough into an 8-inch disk and then fold edges towards the center until round.

5. Press dough, add jalapeno peppers, scallions, cheddar cheese, and fold dough one more time into a round, making sure ingredients are well-incorporated; place seam-side on the working surface (you can wear floured gloves at this point to prevent peppers heat from touching your hands). Loosely cup your hands and mold dough into a round shape while moving around. If the dough is too tacky, dust your hands with some flour and mold.

6. Line Benetton basket with its cover or clean napkin and dust with flour. Wrap basket with a large plastic bag and tie tightly to cover basket fully. Let sit in the room for 1 hour, then refrigerate for 12 to 24 hours.

7. After, fix the oven's rack in the middle and sit a cake pan at the oven's bottom. Pour 3 cups of water into the cake pan and place the Benetton basket on the rack, and let the dough double in size for 2 to 3 hours.

8. Remove basket and cake pan with water. Cut out a 12 x 12-inch greaseproof paper and spray with cooking spray. Unwrap basket, uncover lid, and dust top of the dough with flour.

9. Lay the oiled side of the paper over the dough and inverted the basket onto the counter. Lift basket, cloth, and use a sharp knife to make a ½-inch deep "X" cut into the dough.

10. Pick up the dough while holding edges of parchment paper and lower into Dutch oven.

11. Heat oven to 425ºF and bake bread for 30 minutes once the oven is on. Uncover the pot and bake bread further for 20 to 30 minutes or until deep brown.

12. When ready, carefully remove the hot pot, transfer bread to a wire rack, and let it completely cool for 2 hours.

13. Slice and enjoy bread afterward.

Nutrition:

Calories 110

Carbs 23 g

Fat 0 g

Protein 4 g

77. Beer And Rye Sourdough Bread

Preparation Time: 45 minutes

Cooking Time: 60 minutes

Servings: 8

Ingredients:

- 5 ounces rye flour
- 12 ounces white bread flour + extra for dusting
- 12 ounces beer, room temperature
- 1 tbsps. honey
- 8 ounces sourdough starter
- 1 ¾ tsp. salt

Directions:

1. In a medium bowl, mix flour, water, and sourdough starter until sticky dough forms. Cover bowl with a plastic wrap and let sit at room temperature for 20 minutes.

2. After, remove plastic wrap and sprinkle salt on top; knead the dough until well incorporated. Cover again with a plastic wrap and let rise at room temperature for 30 minutes. Remove wrap after.

3. Holding two edges of the dough with your fingertips, fold the dough over itself into the center. Turn bowl to a 45-degree angle, fold again and repeat this process six more times. Cover the dough and let rise. Repeat folding dough at 30 minute-intervals three more times.

4. Dust a clean, flat working surface with flour. After the fourth and final fold, transfer dough to the surface. Gently spread the dough into an 8-inch disk and then fold edges towards the center until round.

5. Press dough, add jalapeno peppers, scallions, cheddar cheese, and fold dough one more time into a round, making sure ingredients are well-incorporated; place seam-side on the working surface (you can wear floured gloves at this point to prevent peppers heat from touching your hands). Loosely cup your hands and mold dough into a round shape while moving around. If the dough is too tacky, dust your hands with some flour and mold.

6. Line Benetton basket with its cover or clean napkin and dust with flour. Wrap basket with a large plastic bag and tie tightly to cover basket fully. Let sit in the room for 1 hour, then refrigerate for 12 to 24 hours.

7. After, fix the oven's rack in the middle and sit a cake pan at the oven's bottom. Pour 3 cups of water into the cake pan and place the Benetton basket on the rack, and let dough double in size for 2 to 3 hours.

8. Remove basket and cake pan with water. Cut out a 12 x 12-inch greaseproof paper and spray with cooking spray. Unwrap basket, uncover lid, and dust top of the dough with flour.

9. Lay the oiled side of the paper over the dough and inverted the basket onto the counter. Lift basket, cloth, and use a sharp knife to make a ½-inch deep "X" cut into the dough.

10. Pick up the dough while holding edges of parchment paper and lower into Dutch oven.

11. Heat oven to 425ºF and bake bread for 30 minutes once the oven is on. Uncover the pot and bake bread further for 20 to 30 minutes or until deep brown.

12. When ready, carefully remove the hot pot, transfer bread to a wire rack, and let it completely cool for 2 hours.

13. Slice and enjoy bread afterward.

Nutrition:

Calories 110

Carbs 23 g

Fat 0 g

Protein 4 g

78. Blueberry And Lemon Sourdough Bread

Preparation Time: 45 minutes

Cooking Time: 60 minutes

Servings: 8

Ingredients:

- *15 ½ ounces all-purpose flour + extra for dusting*
- 10 ounces water, room temperature
- 8 ounces sourdough starter
- 1 ¾ tsp. salt
- 1 ½ cups fresh blueberries
- 3 lemons, zester

Directions:

1. In a medium bowl, mix flour, water, and sourdough starter until sticky dough forms. Cover bowl with a plastic wrap and let sit at room temperature for 20 minutes.

2. After, remove plastic wrap and sprinkle salt on top; knead the dough until well incorporated. Cover again with a plastic wrap and let rise at room temperature for 30 minutes. Remove wrap after.

3. Holding two edges of the dough with your fingertips, fold the dough over itself into the center. Turn bowl to a 45-degree angle, fold again and repeat this process six more times. Cover the dough and let rise. Repeat folding dough at 30 minute-intervals three more times.

4. Dust a clean, flat working surface with flour. After the fourth and final fold, transfer dough to the surface. Gently spread dough into an 8-inch disk and then fold edges towards the center until round.

5. Press dough, add jalapeno peppers, scallions, cheddar cheese, and fold dough one more time into a round, making sure ingredients are well-incorporated; place seam-side on the working surface (you can wear floured gloves at this point to prevent peppers heat from touching your hands). Loosely cup your

hands and mold dough into a round shape while moving around. If the dough is too tacky, dust your hands with some flour and mold.

6. Line Benetton basket with its cover or clean napkin and dust with flour. Wrap basket with a large plastic bag and tie tightly to cover basket fully. Let sit in the room for 1 hour, then refrigerate for 12 to 24 hours.

7. After, fix the oven's rack in the middle and sit a cake pan at the oven's bottom. Pour 3 cups of water into the cake pan and place the Benetton basket on the rack, and let the dough double in size for 2 to 3 hours.

8. Remove basket and cake pan with water. Cut out a 12 x 12-inch greaseproof paper and spray with cooking spray. Unwrap basket, uncover lid, and dust top of the dough with flour.

9. Lay the oiled side of the paper over the dough and invert the basket onto the counter. Lift basket, cloth, and use a sharp knife to make a ½-inch deep "X" cut into the dough.

10. Pick up the dough while holding edges of parchment paper and lower into Dutch oven.

11. Heat oven to 425ºF and bake bread for 30 minutes once the oven is on. Uncover the pot and bake bread further for 20 to 30 minutes or until deep brown.

12. When ready, carefully remove the hot pot, transfer bread to a wire rack, and let it completely cool for 2 hours.

13. Slice and enjoy bread afterward.

Nutrition:

Calories 110

Carbs 23 g

Fat 0 g

Protein 4 g

Chapter 10. Spice & Herb Breads

79. Original Italian Herb Bread

Preparation Time: 15 minutes

Cooking Time: 3 hours

Servings: 20 slices

Ingredients:

- cup water at 80 degrees F
- ½ cup olive brine
- 1½ tablespoons butter
- tablespoons sugar
- teaspoons salt
- 1/3 cups flour
- 2 teaspoons bread machine yeast
- 20 olives, black/green
- 1½ teaspoons Italian herbs

Directions:

1. Cut olives into slices.
2. Put all ingredients into your bread machine (except olives), carefully following the manufacturer's instructions.
3. Set the program of your bread machine to French bread and set crust type to Medium.
4. Once the maker beeps, add olives.
5. Wait until the cycle completes.
6. Once the loaf is ready, take the bucket out and cool the loaf for 6 minutes.
7. Wobble the bucket to take off the loaf.

Nutrition:

Total Carbs: 71g

Fiber: 1g

Protein: 10g

Fat: 7g

Calories: 386

80. Cinnamon & Dried Fruits Bread

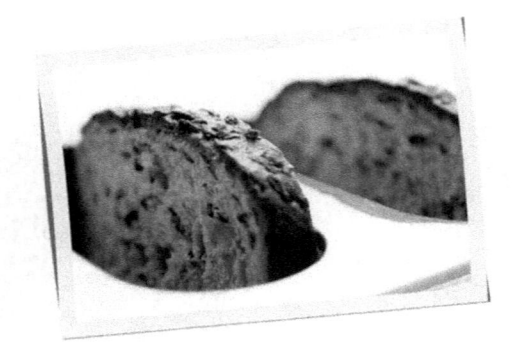

Preparation Time: 5 minutes

Cooking Time: 3 hours

Servings: 16 slices

Ingredients:

- 2¾ cups flour
- 1½ cups of dried fruits
- 4 tablespoons sugar
- 2½ tablespoons butter
- tablespoon milk powder
- teaspoon cinnamon
- ½ teaspoon ground nutmeg
- ¼ teaspoon vanillin
- ½ cup peanuts
- powdered sugar, for sprinkling

- 1 teaspoon salt
- 1½ bread machine yeast

Directions:

1. Mix all of the ingredients to your bread machine (except peanuts and powdered sugar), carefully following the manufacturer's instructions.
2. Set the program of your bread machine to Basic/White Bread and set crust type to Medium.
3. Once the bread maker beeps, moisten dough with a bit of water and add peanuts.
4. Wait until the cycle completes.
5. Once the loaf is ready, take the bucket out and let the loaf cool for a couple of minutes.
6. Shake the bucket to remove the loaf.
7. Sprinkle with powdered sugar.

Nutrition:

Total Carbs: 65g

Fiber: 1g

Protein: 5g

Fat: 4g

Calories: 315

81. Herbal Garlic Cream Cheese Delight

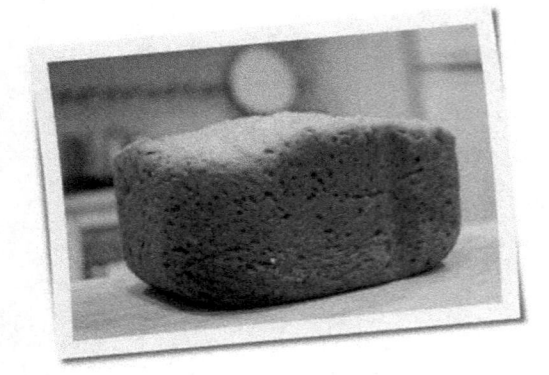

Preparation Time: 5 minutes

Cooking Time: 2 hours and 45 minutes

Servings: 8 slices

Ingredients:

- 1/3 cup water at 80 degrees F
- 1 1/3 cup herb and garlic cream cheese mix, at room temp
- whole egg, beaten, at room temp
- 4 teaspoons melted butter, cooled
- 1 tablespoon sugar
- 2/3 teaspoon salt
- cups white bread flour
- 1 teaspoon instant yeast

Directions:

1. Place all of the ingredients into your device, follow the manufacturer's instructions. Set the program of your bread machine to Basic/White Bread and set crust type to Medium.
2. Wait until the cycle completes.
3. Once the loaf is ready, take the bucket out and let it cool for a couple of minutes.
4. Shake the bucket to remove the loaf.

Nutrition:

Total Carbs: 27g

Fiber: 2g

Protein: 5g

Fat: 6g

Calories: 182

82. Oregano Monza -Cheese Bread

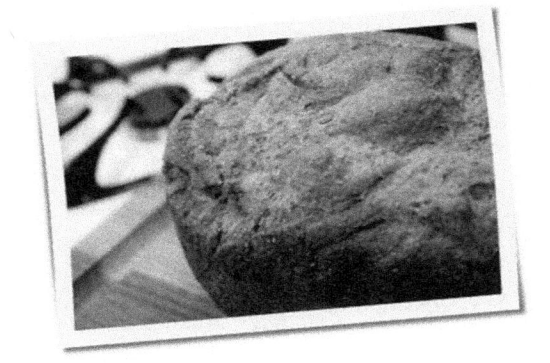

Preparation Time: 15 minutes

Cooking Time: 3 hours and 15 minutes

Servings: 16 slices

Ingredients:

- ½ cup mozzarella cheese
- cup (milk + egg) mixture
- 2¼ cups flour
- ¾ cup whole grain flour
- tablespoons sugar
- 1 teaspoon salt

- teaspoons oregano
- 1½ teaspoons dry yeast

Directions:

1. Place all of the ingredients into your device follow the manufacturer's instructions. Set the program of your bread machine to Basic/White Bread and set crust type to Dark.
2. Wait until the cycle completes.
3. Once the loaf is ready, take the bucket out and let it cool for a couple of minutes.
4. Shake the bucket to remove the loaf.

Nutrition:

Total Carbs: 40g

Fiber: 1g

Protein: 7.7g

Fat: 2.1g

Calories: 209

83. Potato Rosemary Loaf

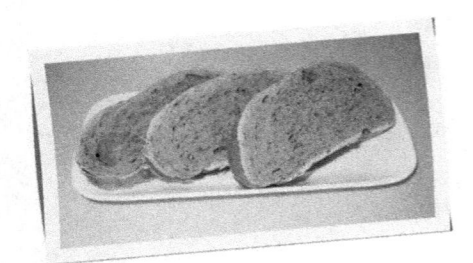

Preparation Time: 5 minutes

Cooking Time: 3 hours and 25 minutes

Servings: 20 slices

Ingredients:

- 4 cups wheat flour
- tablespoon sugar
- 1 tablespoon sunflower oil
- 1½ teaspoons salt
- 1½ cups water
- 1 teaspoon dry yeast
- 1 cup mashed potatoes, ground through a sieve
- crushed rosemary to taste

Directions:

1. Add flour, salt, and sugar to the bread maker bucket and attach the mixing paddle.
2. Add sunflower oil and water.
3. Put in yeast as directed.
4. Set your machine's program to Bread with Filling mode and set crust type to Medium.
5. Once the bread maker beeps and signals to add more ingredients, open the lid, add mashed potatoes, and chopped rosemary.
6. Wait until the cycle completes.
7. Once the loaf is ready, take the bucket out and let the loaf cool for a couple of times.
8. Shake the bucket to remove the loaf.

Nutrition:

Total Carbs: 54g

Fiber: 1g

Protein: 8g

Fat: 3g

Calories: 276

84. Pistachio Cherry Bread

Preparation Time: 5 minutes

Cooking Time: 3 hours and 25 minutes

Servings: 16 slices

Ingredients:

- 1⅛ cups lukewarm water
- 1 egg, at room temperature
- ¼ cup butter, softened
- ¼ cup packed dark brown sugar
- 1½ teaspoons table salt
- 3¾ cups white bread flour
- ½ teaspoon ground nutmeg
- Dash allspice
- 1 teaspoons bread machine yeast
- 1 cup dried cherries
- ½ cup unsalted pistachios, chopped

Directions:

1. Choose the size of the loaf and measure your ingredients.
2. Mix all of the ingredients.
3. Place the pan in the device and close the lid.

4. Select the White/Basic or Fruit/Nut setting, then the loaf size.

5. Add the pistachios and cherries. The machine will automatically add them to the dough during the baking process.

6. When the cycle is processed and the bread is baked, carefully remove the pan from the device.

7. Remove the bread from the device and allow it to cool before slicing.

Nutrition:

Total Carbs: 40g

Fiber: 1g

Protein: 7.7g

Fat: 2.1g

Calories: 209

85. Inspiring Cinnamon Bread

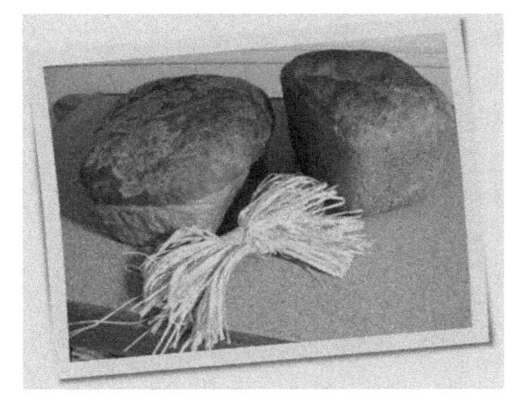

Preparation Time: 15 minutes

Cooking Time: 2 hours and 15 minutes

Servings: 8 slices

Ingredients:

- 2/3 cup milk at 80 degrees F
- whole egg, beaten
- tablespoons melted butter, cooled
- 1/3 cup sugar
- 1/3 teaspoon salt
- 1 teaspoon ground cinnamon
- cups white bread flour
- 1 1/3 teaspoons active dry yeast

Directions:

1. Place all of the ingredients into your device, and follow the manufacturer's instructions.
2. Set the program of your bread machine to Basic/White Bread and set crust type to Medium.
3. Wait until the cycle completes.
4. Once the loaf is ready, take the bucket out and let the loaf cool for 5 minutes.
5. Remove the loaf

Nutrition:

Total Carbs: 34g

Fiber: 1g

Protein: 5g

Fat: 5g

Calories: 198

86. Lavender Buttermilk Bread

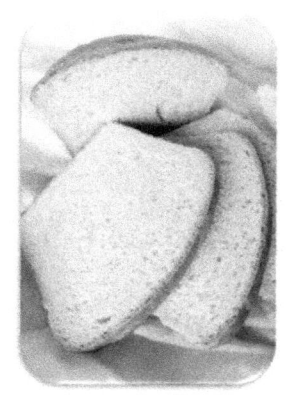

Preparation Time: 10 minutes

Cooking time: 3 hours

Servings: 14

Ingredients:

- ½ cup of water
- 7/8 cup buttermilk
- 1/4 cup olive oil
- 3 Tablespoon finely chopped fresh lavender leaves
- ¼ teaspoon finely chopped fresh lavender flowers
- Grated zest of 1 lemon
- 4 cups bread flour
- teaspoon salt
- 3/4 teaspoon bread machine yeast

Directions:

1. Add each ingredient into the bread machine in the order and at the temperature recommended by your bread machine manufacturer.
2. Close the lid; select the basic bread, medium crust setting on your bread machine, and press start.
3. When the bread machine has finished baking, remove the bread, and put it on a cooling rack.

Nutrition:

Carbs: 27 g

Fat: 5 g

Protein: 2 g

Calories: 170

87. Cardamom Cranberry Bread

Preparation Time: 5 Minutes

Cooking Time: 3 Hours

Servings: 14 slices

Ingredients:

- 1¾ cups water
- 2 Tbsp. brown sugar
- 1½ tsp. salt
- 2 Tbsp. coconut oil
- 4 cups flour
- 2 tsp. cinnamon
- 2 tsp. Cardamom
- cup dried cranberries
- 1 tsp. yeast

Directions:

1. Add each ingredient except the dried cranberries to the bread machine in the order and at the temperature recommended by your bread machine manufacturer.

2. Close the lid; select the basic bread setting on your bread machine and press start.
3. Add the dried cranberries 5 to 10 minutes before the last kneading cycle ends.
4. When the bread machine has stopped baking, remove the bread and put it on a cooling rack.

Nutrition:

Carbs – 41 G

Fat – 3 G

Protein – 3 G

Calories – 157

88. Sesame French Bread

Preparation Time: 20 Minutes

Cooking Time: 3 Hours and 15 Minutes

Servings: 14 slices

Ingredients:

- 7/8 cup water
- 1 tbsp. butter, softened cups
- 1 cup of bread flour
- ½ tsp. sugar
- 1 tsp. salt
- 2 tsp. yeast
- 2 tbsp. sesame seeds toasted

Directions:

1. Add each ingredient to the bread machine in the order and at the temperature indorsed by your bread machine manufacturer.

2. Close the lid; select the French bread, medium crust setting on your bread machine, and press start.
3. When the bread machine has finished baking, remove the bread and put it on a cooling rack.

Nutrition:

Carbs – 28 G

Fat – 3 G

Protein – 6 G

Calories – 160

89. Zucchini Bread

Preparation Time: 15 Minutes |
Cooking Time: 3 Hours 40 Minutes
Servings: 12
Ingredients:
- 1/2 teaspoon salt
- 1 cup of sugar
- 1 tablespoon pumpkin pie spice
- 1 tablespoon baking powder
- 1 teaspoon pure vanilla extract
- 1/3 cup milk
- 1/2 cup vegetable oil
- 2 eggs
- 2 cups bread flour
- 1 1/2 teaspoons bread machine yeast
- 1 cup shredded zucchini, raw and unpeeled
- 1 cup of chopped walnuts (optional)

Directions:

1. Add all of the ingredients for the zucchini bread into the bread maker pan in the order listed above, reserving yeast.
2. Mix all the ingredients and add the yeast.
3. Select the Wheat bread cycle, medium crust color, and press Start.
4. Let it cool before slicing to serve.

Nutrition:

Total Carbs: 54g

Fiber: 1g

Protein: 8g

Fat: 3g

Calories: 276

90. Banana Split Loaf

Preparation Time: 10 Minutes
Cooking Time: 1 Hour
Servings: 12
Ingredients:

- 2 eggs
- 1/3 cup butter, melted
- 2 tablespoons whole milk
- 2 overripe bananas, mashed
- 2 cups all-purpose flour
- 2/3 cups sugar
- 1 1/4 teaspoons baking powder
- 1/2 teaspoon baking soda
- 1/2 teaspoon salt
- 1 cup chopped walnuts

- 1/2 cup chocolate chips

Directions:

1. Pour eggs, butter, milk, and bananas into the bread maker pan and set aside.
2. Add dry ingredients to the bread maker pan.
3. Set to the Basic setting, medium crust color, and press Start.
4. Remove the bread and place it on a cooling rack before serving.

Nutrition:

Calories: 260

Sodium: 203 mg

Dietary Fiber: 1.6 g

Fat: 11.3 g

Carbs: 35.9 g

Protein: 5.2 g.

91. Cranberry Orange Pecan Bread

Preparation Time: 5 Minutes
Cooking Time: 2 Hours 50 Minutes
Servings: 16
Ingredients:

- 1 Cup Water
- 1/4 Cup Orange Juice
- 2 Teaspoons Salt
- 1/3 Cup Sugar
- 2 1/2 Tablespoons Nonfat Dry Milk
- 2 1/2 Tablespoons Butter, Cubed
- 4 Cup Bread Flour
- 2 1/2 Teaspoons Orange Zest

- 2 1/2 Teaspoons Bread Machine Yeast
- 1/2 Cup Dried Cranberries
- 1/2 Cup Pecans, Chopped

Directions:

1. Set aside cranberries and pecans, and then place all other ingredients in the bread maker pan in the order listed.
2. Choose Sweet cycle, light crust, and press Start.
3. Add cranberries and pecans at the end of the kneading cycle.
4. Transfer to a plate and let cool 10 minutes before slicing with a bread knife.

Nutrition:

Total Carbs: 54g

Fiber: 1g

Protein: 8g

Fat: 3g

Calories: 276

92. Caramelized Onion Bread

Preparation Time: 15 Minutes

Cooking Time: 3 Hours and 35 Minutes

Servings: 14 slices

Ingredients:

- ½ Tbsp. butter
- ½ cup onions, sliced
- cup of water
- 1 Tbsp. olive oil
- cups Gold Medal Better

- 1 tsp. salt
- 1¼ tsp. quick active dry yeast

Directions:

1. Melt the butter through medium-low heat in a skillet.
2. Cook the onions in the butter for 10 to 15 minutes until they are brown and caramelized - then remove from the heat.
3. Add each ingredient except the onions to the bread machine.
4. Select the basic bread, medium crust setting on your bread machine, and press start.
5. Add ½ cup of onions 5 to 10 minutes before the last kneading cycle ends.
6. When the bread machine has ended baking, remove the bread and put it on a cooling rack.

Nutrition:

Carbs – 30 G

Fat – 3 G

Protein – 4 G

Calories – 160

93.   Romano Oregano Bread

Preparation Time: 15 minutes

Cooking Time: 3 hours

Servings: 20 slices

Ingredients:

- 16 slice bread (2 pounds)
- 1⅓ cups lukewarm water

- ¼ cup of sugar
- 2 tablespoons olive oil
- 1⅓ teaspoons table salt
- 1⅓ tablespoons dried leaf oregano
- ⅔ cup cheese (Romano or Parmesan), freshly grated
- 4 cups white bread flour
- 2½–3 teaspoons bread machine yeast

- 12 slice bread (1½ pounds)
- 1 cup lukewarm water
- 3 tablespoons sugar
- 1½ tablespoons olive oil
- 1 teaspoon table salt
- 1 tablespoon dried leaf oregano
- ½ cup cheese (Romano or Parmesan), freshly grated
- 3 cups white bread flour
- 2 teaspoons bread machine yeast

Directions:

1. Measure your ingredients for the size of the loaf you would like to make.
2. Place the ingredients into the bread pan.
3. Select the Basic setting, then the loaf size, and finally, the crust color, press start.
4. Remove the pan from the device when the cycle is done,
5. Allow it to cool down before slicing.

Nutrition: per slice

Calories: 207,

Fat: 6.2 g,

Carbs: 27 g,

Sodium: 267 mg,

Protein: 9.3 g

94. Parsley Garlic Bread

Preparation Time: 15 minutes

Cooking Time: 3 hours

Servings: 20 slices

Ingredients:

- 16 slice bread (2 pounds)
- 1⅓ cups lukewarm milk
- 2 tablespoons unsalted butter, melted
- 4 teaspoons sugar
- 2 teaspoons table salt
- 2⅔ teaspoons garlic powder
- 2⅔ teaspoons fresh parsley, chopped
- 4 cups white bread flour
- 2¼ teaspoons bread machine yeast

- 12 slice bread (1½ pounds)
- 1 cup lukewarm milk
- 1½ tablespoons unsalted butter, melted
- 1 tablespoon sugar
- 1½ teaspoons table salt
- 2 teaspoons garlic powder
- 2 teaspoons fresh parsley, chopped
- 3 cups white bread flour
- 1¾ teaspoons bread machine yeast

Directions:

1. Measure your ingredients for the size of the loaf you would like to make.
2. Place the ingredients in the bread pan
3. Select the Basic or Fruit/Nut, then the loaf size, and finally the crust color. Start the cycle.
4. When the device signals to add ingredients, add the toasted pecans.
5. When the cycle is finished, remove the pan from the device
6. Allow it to cool on a wire rack for at least 10 minutes before slicing.

Nutrition:

Total Carbs: 71g

Fiber: 1g

Protein: 10g

Fat: 7g

Calories: 386

95. Swiss Olive Bread

Preparation Time: 5 minutes

Cooking Time: 3 hours

Servings: 16 slices

Ingredients:

- 16 slice bread (2 pounds)
- 1⅓ cups lukewarm milk
- 2 tablespoons unsalted butter, melted
- 1⅓ teaspoons minced garlic
- 2 tablespoons sugar
- 1⅓ teaspoons table salt

- 1 cup Swiss cheese, shredded
- 4 cups white bread flour
- 1½ teaspoons bread machine yeast
- ½ cup chopped black olives
- 12 slice bread (1½ pounds)
- 1 cup lukewarm milk
- 1½ tablespoons unsalted butter, melted
- 1 teaspoon minced garlic
- 1½ tablespoons sugar
- 1 teaspoon table salt
- ¾ cup Swiss cheese, shredded
- 3 cups white bread flour
- 1 teaspoon bread machine yeast
- ⅓ cup chopped black olives

Directions:

1. Measure your ingredients for the size of the loaf you would like to make.
2. Place the ingredients into the bread pan
3. Select the Basic or Fruit/Nut, then the loaf size, and finally the crust color. Start the cycle.
4. When the device signals to add ingredients, add the olives.
5. When the cycle is finished, remove the pan from the device
6. Allow it to cool on a wire rack for at least 10 minutes before slicing.

Nutrition:

Calories 147,

Fat: 4.8 g,

Carbs: 26.7 g,

Sodium: 263 mg,

Protein: 5.8 g

96. Super Spice Bread

Preparation Time: 15 minutes

Cooking Time: 3 hours

Servings: 20 slices

Difficulty: Intermediate

Ingredients:

- 16 slice bread (2 pounds)
- 1⅓ cups lukewarm milk
- 2 eggs, at room temperature
- 2 tablespoons unsalted butter, melted
- 2⅔ tablespoons honey
- 1⅓ teaspoons table salt
- 4 cups white bread flour
- 1⅓ teaspoons ground cinnamon
- ⅔ teaspoon ground cardamom
- ⅔ teaspoon ground nutmeg
- 2¼ teaspoons bread machine yeast
- 12 slice bread (1½ pounds)
- 1 cup lukewarm milk
- 2 eggs, at room temperature
- 1½ tablespoons unsalted butter, melted
- 2 tablespoons honey
- 1 teaspoon table salt
- 3 cups white bread flour
- 1 teaspoon ground cinnamon
- ½ teaspoon ground cardamom
- ½ teaspoon ground nutmeg
- 2 teaspoons bread machine yeast

Directions:

1. Measure your ingredients for the size of the loaf you would like to make.
2. Place the ingredients into the bread pan
3. Select the Basic or Fruit/Nut, then the loaf size, and finally the crust color. Start the cycle.
4. When the device signals to add ingredients, add the toasted pecans.
5. When the cycle is finished, remove the pan from the device
6. Allow it to cool on a wire rack for at least 10 minutes before slicing.

Nutrition:

Calories: 163,

Fat: 2.8 g,

Carbs: 27.6 g,

Sodium: 97 mg,

Protein: 4.8 g

97. Anise Honey Bread

Preparation Time: 15 minutes

Cooking Time: 3 hours

Servings: 20 slices

Ingredients:

- 16 slice bread (2 pounds)
- 1 cup + 1 tablespoon lukewarm water
- 1 egg, at room temperature
- ⅓ cup butter, melted and cooled
- ⅓ cup honey
- ⅔ teaspoon table salt

- 4 cups white bread flour
- 1⅓ teaspoons anise seed
- 1⅓ teaspoons lemon zest
- 2½ teaspoons bread machine yeast
- 12 slice bread (1½ pounds)
- ¾ cup lukewarm water
- 1 egg, at room temperature
- ¼ cup butter, melted and cooled
- ¼ cup honey
- ½ teaspoon table salt
- 3 cups white bread flour
- 1 teaspoon anise seed
- 1 teaspoon lemon zest
- 2 teaspoons bread machine yeast

Directions:

1. Measure your ingredients for the size of the loaf you would like to make.
2. Place the ingredients into the bread pan.
3. Select the Basic setting, then the loaf size, and finally, the crust color, press start.
4. When the cycle is finished, remove the pan from the device
5. Allow it to cool on a wire rack for at least 10 minutes before slicing.

Nutrition:

Calories 157,

Fat: 4.8 g,

Carbs: 29.6 g

Sodium: 134 mg,

Protein: 4.7 g

98. Basic Pecan Bread

Preparation Time: 15 minutes

Cooking Time: 3 hours

Servings: 20 slices

Ingredients:

- 16 slice bread (2 pounds)
- 1⅓ cups lukewarm milk
- 2⅔ tablespoons unsalted butter, melted
- 1 egg, at room temperature
- 2⅔ tablespoons sugar
- 1⅓ teaspoons table salt
- 4 cups white bread flour
- 2 teaspoons bread machine yeast
- 1⅓ cups chopped pecans, toasted
- 12 slice bread (1½ pounds)
- 1 cup lukewarm milk
- 2 tablespoons unsalted butter, melted
- 1 egg, at room temperature
- 2 tablespoons sugar
- 1 teaspoon table salt
- 3 cups white bread flour
- 1½ teaspoons bread machine yeast
- 1 cup chopped pecans, toasted

Directions:

7. Measure your ingredients for the size of the loaf you would like to make.
8. Place the ingredients in the bread pan
9. Select the Basic or Fruit/Nut, then the loaf size, and finally the crust color. Start the cycle.
10. When the device signals to add ingredients, add the toasted pecans.

11. When the cycle is finished, remove the pan from the device
12. Allow it to cool on a wire rack for at least 10 minutes before slicing.

Nutrition:

Calories: 168,

Fat: 4.8 g,

Carbs: 25.6 g,

Sodium: 217 mg,

Protein: 5 g

Chapter 11. Nut Breads

99. Cranberry Walnut Wheat Bread

Preparation Time: 15 Minutes |

Cooking Time: 3 Hours 30 Minutes

Servings: 12

Ingredients:

- 1 cup of warm water
- 1 tablespoon molasses
- 2 tablespoons butter
- 1 teaspoon salt
- 2 cups 100% whole wheat flour
- 1 cup unbleached flour
- 2 tablespoons dry milk
- 1 cup cranberries
- 1 cup walnuts, chopped
- 2 teaspoons active dry yeast

Directions:

1. Add the liquid ingredients to the bread maker pan.
2. Add the dry ingredients, except the yeast, walnuts, and cranberries.
3. Make out a well in the center of the bread flour and add the yeast.
4. Insert the pan into your bread maker and secure the lid.
5. Select Wheat Bread setting, choose your preferred crust color, and press Start.
6. Add cranberries and walnuts after the first kneading cycle is finished.
7. Take out the bread from the oven and let it cool before slicing.

Nutrition:

Calories: 126

Sodium: 211 mg

Dietary Fiber: 3.8 g

Fat: 2.6 g

Carbs: 23.2 g

Protein: 4.5 g.

100. Brown Sugar Date Nut Swirl Bread

Preparation Time: 15 Minutes
Cooking Time: 2 Hours 30 Minutes
Servings: 16
Ingredients:

- 1 cup milk
- 1 large egg
- 4 tablespoons butter
- 4 tablespoons sugar
- 1 teaspoon salt
- 4 cups flour
- 1 2/3 teaspoons yeast
- For the filling:
- 1/2 cup packed brown sugar
- 1 cup walnuts, chopped
- 1 cup Medrol dates, pitted and chopped
- 2 teaspoons cinnamon
- 2 teaspoons clove spice
- 1 1/3 tablespoons butter
- Powdered sugar, sifted

Directions:

1. Add wet ingredients to the bread maker pan.
2. Mix flour, sugar, and salt and add to the pan.
3. Make out a well in the center of the dry ingredients and add the yeast.
4. 4Select the Dough cycle and press Start.
5. Smack the dough and allow it to rest in a warm place.
6. Mix the brown sugar with walnuts, dates, and spices; set aside.
7. Baste with a tablespoon of butter, add the filling.
8. Start from the short side and roll the dough to form a jelly roll shape.
9. Let it rise for about 30 minutes.
10. Bake for approximately 30 minutes.
11. Use foil to cover for 10 minutes.
12. Sprinkle with the powdered sugar and serve.

Nutrition:

Total Carbs: 54g

Fiber: 1g

Protein: 8g

Fat: 3g

Calories: 276

101. Raisin Bread

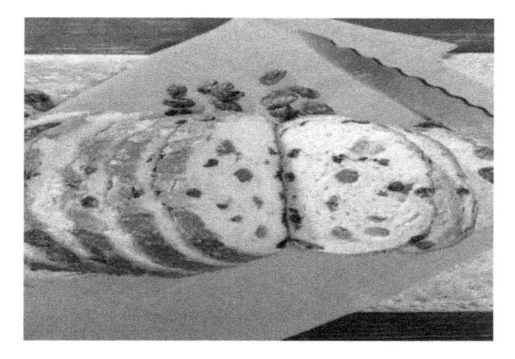

Preparation Time: 5 Minutes
Cooking Time: 3 Hours
Servings: 12
Ingredients:

- 1 cup of warm water
- 3 tablespoons vegetable oil
- 3 cups flour
- 1 teaspoon cinnamon
- 1/8 teaspoon nutmeg
- 1/3 cup sugar
- 1 1/2 teaspoons salt
- 1 packet instant dry yeast
- 3/4 cup raisins

Directions:

1. Add the water and oil to the bread maker.
2. Add flour and sprinkle with cinnamon and nutmeg.
3. On top of the flour, add sugar to one corner of the bread maker, salt in the other corner, and yeast in another corner, so the yeast is not touching sugar and salt.

4. Set to Basic bread cycle, medium crust color, and press Start.

5. Add the raisins when the dough cycle is finished.

6. When the baking process is completed, transfer to a cooling rack for 15 minutes before slicing.

Nutrition:

Calories: 193,

Sodium: 1068 mg,

Dietary Fiber: 1.3 g,

Fat: 3.8 g

Carbs: 36.8 g

Protein: 3.5 g.

102. Multigrain Bread

Preparation Time: 15 Minutes
Cooking Time: 2 Hours 30 Minutes
Servings: 8 slices
Ingredients:

- ¾ cups of water
- 1 tablespoon melted butter, cooled
- ½ tablespoon honey
- ½ teaspoon salt
- ¾ cup multigrain flour
- 1⅓ cups white bread flour
- 1 teaspoon bread machine or active dry yeast

Directions:

1. Place the ingredients in your device.
2. Program the machine for Basic, and press Start.
3. When the loaf is processed, remove the bucket from the device.
4. Let it cool for 20 minutes.
5. Shake the bucket to remove the loaf.

Nutrition:

Calories: 118 calories

Total Carbohydrate: 23.6 g

Cholesterol: 2 g

Total Fat: 1 g

Protein: 4.1 g

Sodium: 304 mg

Sugar: 1.6 g

103. Toasted Pecan Bread

Preparation Time: 15 Minutes
Cooking Time: 2 Hours 30 Minutes
Servings: 8 slices
Ingredients:

- ⅔ cup milk, at 70°F to 80°F
- 4 teaspoons melted butter, cooled
- 1 egg, at room temperature
- 4 teaspoons sugar
- ⅔ teaspoon salt
- 2 cups white bread flour
- 1 teaspoon bread machine or instant yeast

- ⅔ cup chopped pecans, toasted

Directions:

1. Place the ingredients in your device.
2. Program the machine for Basic. Select light, and press Start.
3. When the loaf is processed, remove the bucket from the device.
4. Let it cool for 20 minutes.
5. Shake the bucket to remove the loaf.
6. Let the loaf cool.
7. Slice and serve

Nutrition:

Calories: 126

Sodium: 211 mg

Dietary Fiber: 3.8 g

Fat: 2.6 g

Carbs: 23.2 g

Protein: 4.5 g.

104. Market Seed Bread

Preparation Time: 15 Minutes
Cooking Time: 2 Hours 30 Minutes
Servings: 8 slices
Ingredients:

- ¾ cup milk
- 1 tablespoon melted butter, cooled
- 1 tablespoon honey
- ½ teaspoon salt
- 2 tablespoons flaxseed
- 2 tablespoons sesame seeds

- 1 tablespoon poppy seeds
- ¾ cup whole-wheat flour
- 1¼ cups white bread flour
- 1¼ teaspoons yeast

Directions:

1. Place the ingredients in your device.
2. Program the machine for Basic. Select light or medium crust, and press Start.
3. When the loaf is processed, remove the bucket from the device.
4. Let it cool for 20 minutes.
5. Shake the bucket to remove the loaf.

Nutrition:

Calories: 126

Sodium: 211 mg

Dietary Fiber: 3.8 g

Fat: 2.6 g

Carbs: 23.2 g

Protein: 4.5 g.

107. Hazelnut Honey Bread

Preparation Time: 15 Minutes
Cooking Time: 2 Hours 30 Minutes
Servings: 8 slices
Ingredients:

- 1 cup lukewarm milk
- 2 egg, at room temperature
- 3¾ tablespoons unsalted butter, melted

- 1 tablespoons honey
- ¾ teaspoon pure vanilla extract
- ¾ teaspoon table salt
- 2cups white bread flour
- ¾ cup toasted hazelnuts, finely ground

Directions:

1. Choose the size of loaf and measure the ingredients.
2. Group the ingredients to the bread pan.
3. Place the pan in the device and close the lid.
4. Turn on the bread maker. Select the White/Basic setting, start the cycle.
5. When the cycle is processed and the bread is baked, remove the pan from the device. Let rest for a few minutes.
6. Allow it to cool before slicing.

Nutrition:

Calories: 118 calories

Total Carbohydrate: 23.6 g

Cholesterol: 2 g

Total Fat: 1 g

Protein: 4.1 g

Sodium: 304 mg

Sugar: 1.6 g

108. Double Coconut Bread

Preparation Time: 15 Minutes

Cooking Time: 2 Hours 30 Minutes

Servings: 16 slices

Ingredients:

- 11/4 cup of milk
- 1 egg
- 2 tablespoons melted butter, cooled
- 2⅔ teaspoons pure coconut extract
- 3⅓ tablespoons sugar
- 1 teaspoon salt
- ⅔ cup sweetened shredded coconut
- 4 tablespoon white bread flour
- 2 teaspoons instant yeast

Directions:

1. Place the ingredients in your device.
2. Program the machine for Sweetbread. Select light or medium crust, and press Start.
3. When the loaf is processed, remove the bucket from the device.
4. Let it cool for 20 minutes.
5. Shake the bucket to remove the loaf.

Nutrition:

Calories: 183 calories

Total Carbohydrate: 28 g

Total Fat: 4g

Protein: 6 g

Sodium: 344 mg

109. Flax And Sunflower Seed Bread

Preparation Time: 5 Minutes

Cooking Time: 25 Minutes

Servings: 8

Ingredients:

- 1 1/3 cups water
- 2 tablespoons butter softened
- 3 tablespoons honey
- 2/3 cups of bread flour
- 1 teaspoon salt
- 1 teaspoon active dry yeast
- 1/2 cup flax seeds
- 1/2 cup sunflower seeds

Directions:

1. With the manufacturer's suggested order, add all the ingredients (apart from sunflower seeds) to the bread machine's pan.
2. The select basic white cycle, then press starts.
3. Just in the knead cycle that your machine signals alert sounds, add the sunflower seeds.

Nutrition:

Calories: 140 calories;

Sodium: 169

Total Carbohydrate: 22.7

Cholesterol: 4

Protein: 4.2

Total Fat: 4.2

110. Honey And Flaxseed Bread

Preparation Time: 5 Minutes

Cooking Time: 25 Minutes

Servings: 8

Ingredients:

- 1 1/8 cups water
- 1 1/2 tablespoons flaxseed oil
- 3 tablespoons honey
- 1/2 tablespoon liquid lecithin
- 3 cups whole wheat flour
- 1/2 cup flax seed
- 2 tablespoons bread flour
- 3 tablespoons whey powder
- 1 1/2 teaspoons sea salt
- Two teaspoons active dry yeast

Directions:

1. In the bread machine pan, put in all of the ingredients following the order recommended by the manufacturer.
2. Choose the Wheat cycle on the machine and press the Start button to run the machine.

Nutrition:

Calories: 174 calories;

Protein: 7.1

Total Fat: 4.9

Sodium: 242

Total Carbohydrate: 30.8

Cholesterol: 1

111. Pumpkin And Sunflower Seed Bread

Preparation Time: 5 Minutes

Cooking Time: 25 Minutes

Servings: 8

Ingredients:

- 1 (.25 ounce) package instant yeast
- 1 cup of warm water
- 1/4 cup honey
- 4 teaspoons vegetable oil
- 3 cups whole wheat flour
- 1/4 cup wheat bran (optional)
- 1 teaspoon salt
- 1/3 cup sunflower seeds
- 1/3 cup shelled, toasted, chopped pumpkin seeds

Directions:

1. Into the bread machine, put the ingredients according to the order suggested by the manufacturer.
2. Next is setting the device to the whole wheat setting, then press the start button.
3. You can add the pumpkin and sunflower seeds at the beep if your bread machine has a signal for nuts or fruit.

Nutrition:

Calories: 148 calories;

Total Carbohydrate: 24.1

Cholesterol: 0

Protein: 5.1

Total Fat: 4.8

Sodium: 158

112. Seven Grain Bread

Preparation Time: 5 Minutes
Cooking Time: 25 Minutes
Servings: 8
Ingredients:
- 1 1/3 cups warm water
- 1 tablespoon active dry yeast
- 3 tablespoons dry milk powder
- 2 tablespoons vegetable oil
- 2 tablespoons honey
- 2 teaspoons salt
- 1 egg
- 1 cup whole wheat flour
- 2 1/2 cups bread flour
- 3/4 cup 7-grain cereal

Directions:
1. Follow the order of putting the ingredients into the pan of the bread machine recommended by the manufacturer.
2. Choose the Whole Wheat Bread cycle on the device and press the Start button to run the machine.

Nutrition:

Calories: 285 calories;

Total Fat: 5.2

Sodium: 629

Total Carbohydrate: 50.6

Cholesterol: 24

Protein: 9.8

113. Wheat Bread With Flax Seed

Preparation Time: 5 Minutes

Cooking Time: 25 Minutes

Servings: 8

Ingredients:

- 1 package active dry yeast
- 1 1/4 cups whole wheat flour
- 3/4 cup ground flax seed
- 1 cup bread flour
- 1 tablespoon vital wheat gluten
- 2 tablespoons dry milk powder
- 1 teaspoon salt
- 1 1/2 tablespoons vegetable oil
- 1/4 cup honey
- 1 1/2 cups water

Directions:

1. In the bread machine pan, put the ingredients following the order recommendation of the manufacturer.
2. Make sure to select the cycle and then press Start.

Nutrition:

Calories: 168 calories

Total Carbohydrate: 22.5

Cholesterol: 1

Protein: 5.5

Total Fat: 7.3

Sodium: 245

114. High Fiber Bread

Preparation Time: 5 Minutes

Cooking Time: 25 Minutes

Servings: 8

Ingredients:

- 1 2/3 cups warm water
- Four teaspoons molasses
- One tablespoon active dry yeast
- 2 2/3 cups whole wheat flour
- 3/4 cup ground flax seed
- 2/3 cup bread flour
- 1/2 cup oat bran
- 1/3 cup rolled oats
- 1/3 cup amaranth seeds
- One teaspoon salt

Directions:

1. In the bread machine pan, put in the water, molasses, yeast, wheat flour, ground flaxseed, bread flour, oat bran, rolled oats, amaranth seeds, and salt in the manufacturer's suggested order of ingredients. Choose the Dough cycle on the machine and press the Start button; let the machine finish the whole Dough cycle.
2. Put the dough on a clean surface that is covered with a little bit of flour. Use a slightly wet cloth to shelter the loaves and allow them to rise.
3. Preheat the oven to 375°F.

4. Put in the warm-up oven and bake for 20-25 minutes until the top part of the loaf turns golden brown. Let the loaf slide onto a clean working surface and tap the loaf's bottom part gently. The bread is done if you hear a hollow sound when tapped.

Nutrition:

Calories: 101 calories;

Total Fat: 2.1

Sodium: 100

Total Carbohydrate: 18.2

Cholesterol: 0

Protein: 4

115. High Flavor Bran Head

Preparation Time: 5 Minutes

Cooking Time: 25 Minutes

Servings: 8

Ingredients:

- 1 1/2 cups warm water
- Two tablespoons dry milk powder
- Two tablespoons vegetable oil
- Two tablespoons molasses
- Two tablespoons honey
- 1 1/2 teaspoons salt
- 2 1/4 cups whole wheat flour
- 1 1/4 cups bread flour
- 1 cup whole bran cereal

- Two teaspoons active dry yeast

Directions:

1. In the pan of your bread machine, move all the ingredients directed by the machine's maker.
2. Set the device to either the whole grain or whole wheat setting.

Nutrition:

Calories: 146 calories

Total Fat: 2.4

Sodium: 254

Total Carbohydrate: 27.9

Cholesterol: 1

Protein: 4.6

116. High Protein Bread

Preparation Time: 5 Minutes

Cooking Time: 25 Minutes

Servings: 8

Ingredients:

- Two teaspoons active dry yeast
- 1 cup bread flour
- 1 cup whole wheat flour
- 1/4 cup soy flour
- 1/4 cup powdered soy milk
- 1/4 cup oat bran
- One tablespoon canola oil
- One tablespoon honey

- One teaspoon salt
- 1 cup of water

Directions:

1. Into the bread machine's pan, put the ingredients by following the order suggested by the manufacturer.
2. Set the device to either the regular setting or the primary medium.
3. Push the Start button.

Nutrition:

Calories: 137 calories

Total Fat: 2.4

Sodium: 235

Total Carbohydrate: 24.1

Cholesterol: 0

Protein: 6.5

117. Whole Wheat Bread With Sesame Seeds

Preparation Time: 5 Minutes

Cooking Time: 25 Minutes

Servings: 8

Ingredients:

- 1/2 cup water
- 2 teaspoons honey
- 1 tablespoon vegetable oil
- 3/4 cup grated zucchini
- 3/4 cup whole wheat flour
- 2 cups bread flour

- 1 tablespoon chopped fresh basil
- 2 teaspoons sesame seeds
- 1 teaspoon salt
- 1 ½ teaspoon active dry yeast

Directions:

1. Follow the order of putting the ingredients into the bread machine pan recommended by the manufacturer.
2. Choose the Basic Bread cycle or the Normal setting on the machine.

Nutrition:

Calories: 153 calories

Sodium: 235

Total Carbohydrate: 28.3

Cholesterol: 0

Protein: 5

Total Fat: 2.3

118. Bagels With Poppy Seeds

Preparation Time: 5 Minutes

Cooking Time: 25 Minutes

Servings: 8

Ingredients:

- 1 cup of warm water
- 1 1/2 teaspoons salt
- 2 tablespoons white sugar
- 3 cups bread flour
- 2 1/4 teaspoons active dry yeast

- 3 quarts boiling water
- 3 tablespoons white sugar
- 1 tablespoon cornmeal
- 1 egg white
- 3 tablespoons poppy seeds

Directions:

1. In the bread machine's pan, pour in the water, salt, sugar, flour, and yeast following the order of ingredients suggested by the manufacturer. Choose the Dough setting on the machine.
2. Once the machine has finished the whole cycle, place the dough on a clean surface covered with a little bit of flour; let it rest. While the dough is resting on the floured surface, put 3 quarts of water in a big pot and let it boil. Add in 3 tablespoons of sugar and mix.
3. Divide the dough evenly into nine portions and shape each into a small ball. Press down each dough ball until it is flat. Use your thumb to make a shack in the center of each flattened dough. Increase the whole's size in the center and smoothen out the dough around the whole area by spinning the dough on your thumb or finger. Use a clean cloth to cover the formed bagels and let them sit for 10 minutes.
4. Cover the bottom part of an ungreased baking sheet evenly with cornmeal. Place the bagels gently into the boiling water. Let it boil for 1 minute and flip it on the other side halfway through. Let the bagels drain quickly on a clean towel. Place the boiled bagels onto the prepared baking sheet. Coat the topmost of each bagel with egg white and top it off with your preferred toppings.
5. Put the bagels into the preheated 375°F (190°C) oven and bake for 20-25 minutes until it turns nice brown.

Nutrition:

Calories: 50 calories

Total Fat: 1.3

Sodium: 404

Total Carbohydrate: 8.8

119. Macadamia Nut Bread

Preparation Time: 5 minutes

Cooking Time: 21 min

Servings: 6

Ingredients:

- 5 ounces macadamia nuts I utilized the Royal Hawaiian brand
- 5 enormous eggs
- 1/4 cup coconut flour (28 g)
- 1/2 teaspoon heating pop
- 1/2 teaspoon apple juice vinegar

Directions:

1. Preheat broiler to 350F.
2. To a blender or nourishment processor, include macadamia nuts and heartbeat until it becomes nut margarine. On the off chance that your blender doesn't work superbly without fluid, have eggs each in turn until the consistency is that of nut margarine.
3. Scrape drawbacks of blender or nourishment processor, and include remaining eggs. Mix until well-fused.
4. Add in coconut flour, heating pop, and apple juice vinegar and heartbeat until consolidated.
5. Grease a standard-size bread dish and include the hitter. The hitter's smooth surface and spot-on a base rack of the boiler for 30-40 minutes, or until the top is brilliant dark-colored.
6. Remove from stove and permit to cool in prospect 20 minutes before evacuating.

7. Will store in a water/air proof compartment at room temperature for 3-4 days at room temperature or multi-week in the refrigerator.

Nutrition:

Cal: 40

Carbs: 4g

Net Carbs: 3.5 g

Fiber: 8.5 g

Fat: 14 g

Protein: 10g

120. Paled Coconut Bread

Preparation Time: 12 minutes

Cooking Time: 22 min

Servings: 8

Ingredients:

- 1/2 cup coconut flour
- 1/4 teaspoon salt
- 1/4 teaspoon heating pop
- 6 eggs
- ¼ cup coconut oil, liquefied
- ¼ unsweetened almond milk

Directions:

1. Preheat broiler to 350°F.
2. Line an 8×4 inch portion container with material paper.
3. In a bowl, consolidate the coconut flour, preparing pop and salt.
4. In another bowl, reduce the eggs, milk, and oil.

5. Slowly include the wet fixings into the dry fixings and blend until consolidated.
6. Pour the blend into the readied portion container.
7. Bake for 40-50 minutes, or until a toothpick embedded in the center tells the truth.

Nutrition:

Cal: 40

Carbs: 4g

Net Carbs: 2.5 g

Fiber: 7.5 g

Fat: 12 g

Protein: 6g

Chapter 12. Sweet & Chocolate Bread

121. Currant Bread

Preparation Time: 10 minutes

Cooking time: 3½ hours

Servings: 10

Ingredients:

- 1¼ cups warm milk
- 2 tablespoons light olive oil
- 2 tablespoons maple syrup
- 3 cups bread flour
- 2 teaspoons ground cardamom
- 1 teaspoon salt
- 2 teaspoons active dry yeast
- ½ cup currants
- ½ cup cashews, chopped finely

Directions:

1. Place all ingredients (except for currants and cashews) in the baking pan of the bread machine in the order recommended by the manufacturer.
2. Place the baking pan in the bread machine and close the lid.
3. Select the Basic setting.
4. Press the start button.
5. Wait for the bread machine to beep before adding the currants and cashews.
6. Carefully remove the baking pan from the machine and then invert the bread loaf onto a wire rack to cool completely before slicing.
7. With a sharp knife, cut bread loaf into desired-sized slices and serve.

Nutrition:

Calories 232

Total Fat 7.1 g

Saturated Fat 1.5 g

Cholesterol 3 mg

Sodium 250 mg

Total Carbs 36.4 g

Fiber 1.7 g

Sugar 4.6 g

Protein 6.4 g

122.   Pineapple Juice Bread

Preparation Time: 5 minutes

Cooking time: 3 hours

Servings: 12

Ingredients:

- ¾ cup fresh pineapple juice
- 1 egg
- 2 tablespoons vegetable oil
- 2½ tablespoons honey
- ¾ teaspoon salt
- 3 cups bread flour
- 2 tablespoons dry milk powder
- 2 teaspoons quick-rising yeast

Directions:

1. Place all ingredients in the baking pan of the bread machine in the order recommended by the manufacturer.
2. Place the baking pan in the bread machine and close the lid.

3. Select Sweet Bread setting and then Light Crust.
4. Press the start button.
5. Carefully remove the baking pan from the machine and then invert the bread loaf onto a wire rack to cool completely before slicing.
6. With a sharp knife, cut bread loaf into desired-sized slices and serve.

Nutrition:

Calories 168

Total Fat 3 g

Saturated Fat 0.6 g

Cholesterol 14 mg

Sodium 161 mg

Total Carbs 30.5 g

Fiber 1 g

Sugar 5.9 g

Protein 4.5 g

123. Mocha Bread

Preparation Time: 15 minutes

Cooking time: 30 minutes

Servings: 12

Ingredients:

- 1/8 cup coffee-flavored liqueur
- ¼ cup of water
- 1 (5-ounce) can evaporate milk
- 1 teaspoon salt

- 1½ teaspoons vegetable oil
- 3 cups bread flour
- 2 tablespoons brown sugar
- 1 teaspoon active dry yeast
- ¼ cup semi-sweet mini chocolate chips

Directions:

1. Take all ingredients (except the chocolate chips) in the baking pan of the bread machine in the order recommended by the manufacturer.
2. Place the baking pan in the bread machine and close the lid.
3. Select the Dough cycle.
4. Press the start button.
5. After the Dough cycle completes, remove the dough from the bread pan and place it onto a lightly floured surface.
6. With a plastic wrap, cover the dough for about 10 minutes.
7. Uncover the dough and roll it into a rectangle.
8. Sprinkle the dough with chocolate chips and then shape it into a loaf.
9. Now, place the dough into a greased loaf pan.
10. With a plastic wrap, cover the loaf pan and set in a warm place for 45 minutes or until doubled in size.
11. Preheat your oven to 375ºF.
12. Bake for approximately 24–30 minutes or until a wooden skewer inserted in the center comes out clean.
13. Now, invert bread onto the wire rack to cool completely before slicing.
14. With a sharp knife, cut the bread loaf into desired-sized slices and serve.

Nutrition:

Calories 179

Total Fat 4.6 g

Saturated Fat 1.8 g

Cholesterol 3 mg

Sodium 208 mg

Total Carbs 29.8 g

Fiber 1.2 g

Sugar 5.3 g

Protein 4.2 g

124. Maple Syrup Bread

Preparation Time: 5 minutes

Cooking time: 3 hours

Servings: 12

Ingredients:

- 1 cup buttermilk
- 2 tablespoons maple syrup
- 2 tablespoons vegetable oil
- 2 tablespoons non-fat dry milk powder
- 1 cup whole-wheat flour
- 2 cups bread flour
- 1 teaspoon salt
- 1½ teaspoons bread machine yeast

Directions:

1. Place all ingredients in the baking pan of the bread machine in the order recommended by the manufacturer.
2. Place the baking pan in the bread machine and close the lid.
3. Select the Basic setting.
4. Press the start button.
5. Carefully remove the baking pan from the machine and then invert the bread loaf onto a wire rack to cool completely before slicing.
6. With a sharp knife, cut bread loaf into desired-sized slices and serve.

Nutrition:

Calories 151

Total Fat 2.6 g

Saturated Fat 0.6 g

Cholesterol 1 mg

Sodium 217 mg

Total Carbs 26.1 g

Fiber 0.4 g

Sugar 3.8 g

Protein 4.7 g

125. Peanut Butter & Jelly Bread

Preparation Time: 5 minutes

Cooking time: 3 hours

Servings: 12

Ingredients:

- 1 cup of water
- 1½ tablespoons vegetable oil
- ½ cup peanut butter
- ½ cup blackberry jelly
- 1 tablespoon white sugar
- 1 teaspoon salt
- 1 cup whole-wheat flour
- 2 cups bread flour
- 1½ teaspoons active dry yeast

Directions:

1. Place all ingredients in the baking pan of the bread machine in the order recommended by the manufacturer.

2. Place the baking pan in the bread machine and close the lid.
3. Select Sweet Bread setting.
4. Press the start button.
5. Carefully remove the baking pan from the machine and then invert the bread loaf onto a wire rack to cool completely before slicing.
6. With a sharp knife, cut bread loaf into desired-sized slices and serve.

Nutrition:

Calories 218

Total Fat 7.2 g

Saturated Fat 1.5 g

Cholesterol 0 mg

Sodium 245 mg

Total Carbs 31.6 g

Fiber 1.1 g

Sugar 2.7 g

Protein 6.7 g

126. Brown & White Sugar Bread

Preparation Time: 5 minutes

Cooking time: 2 hours 55 minutes

Servings: 12

Ingredients:

- 1 cup milk (room temperature)
- ¼ cup butter softened
- 1 egg

- ¼ cup light brown sugar
- ¼ cup granulated white sugar
- 2 tablespoons ground cinnamon
- ¼ teaspoon salt
- 3 cups bread flour
- 2 teaspoons bread machine yeast

Directions:

1. Place all ingredients in the baking pan of the bread machine in the order recommended by the manufacturer.
2. Place the baking pan in the bread machine and close the lid.
3. Select Sweet Bread setting and then Medium Crust.
4. Press the start button.
5. Carefully remove the baking pan from the machine and then invert the bread loaf onto a wire rack to cool completely before slicing.
6. With a sharp knife, cut bread loaf into desired-sized slices and serve.

Nutrition:

Calories 195

Total Fat 5 g

Saturated Fat 2.8 g

Cholesterol 25 mg

Sodium 94 mg

Total Carbs 33.2 g

Fiber 1.6 g

Sugar 8.2 g

Protein 4.7 g

127. Molasses Bread

Preparation Time: 5 minutes

Cooking time: 4 hours

Servings: 12

Ingredients:

- 1/3 cup milk
- ¼ cup of water
- 3 tablespoons molasses
- 3 tablespoons butter, softened
- 2 cups bread flour
- 1¾ cups whole-wheat flour
- 2 tablespoons white sugar
- 1 teaspoon salt
- 2¼ teaspoons quick-rising yeast

Directions:

1. Place all ingredients in the baking pan of the bread machine in the order recommended by the manufacturer.
2. Place the baking pan in the bread machine and close the lid.
3. Select Light Browning setting.
4. Press the start button.
5. Carefully remove the baking pan from the machine and then invert the bread loaf onto a wire rack to cool completely before slicing.
6. With a sharp knife, cut bread loaf into desired-sized slices and serve.

Nutrition:

Calories 205

Total Fat 3.9 g

Saturated Fat 1.9 g

Cholesterol 8 mg

Sodium 220 mg

Total Carbs 37.4 g

Fiber 3.1 g

Sugar 5.1 g

Protein 5.6 g

128. Chocolate Zucchini Bread

Preparation Time: 10 minutes

Cooking time: 4 hours

Servings: 14 slices

Ingredients:

- 1 cup / 200 grams grated zucchini, moisture squeezed thoroughly
- 1/3 cup / 60 grams ground flaxseed
- ½ cup / 100 grams almond flour
- ½ teaspoon salt
- 2 ½ teaspoons baking powder
- 1 ¼ tablespoon psyllium husk powder
- 1/3 cup / 60 grams of cocoa powder
- 4 eggs, pasteurized
- 1 tablespoon coconut cream
- 5 tablespoons coconut oil
- ¾ cup / 150 grams erythritol sweetener
- 1 teaspoon vanilla extract, unsweetened
- ½ cup / 115 grams sour cream
- ½ cup / 100 grams chocolate chips, unsweetened

Directions:

1. Wrap zucchini in cheesecloth and twist well until all the moisture is released; set aside until required.
2. Gather all the ingredients for the bread and plug in the bread machine having the capacity of 2 pounds of bread recipe.
3. Take a large bowl, place flaxseed and flour in it, and then stir salt, baking powder, husk, and cocoa powder in it until mixed.
4. Take a separate large bowl, crack eggs in it and then beat in coconut cream, coconut oil, sweetener, and vanilla until combined.
5. Blend the flour mixture, then sour cream and the remaining half of the flour mixture until incorporated. And then fold in chocolate chips until mixed.
6. Add batter into the bread bucket, shut the lid, select the "basic/white" cycle setting and then press the up/down arrow button to adjust baking time according to your bread machine; it will take 3 to 4 hours.
7. Then press the crust button to select light crust if available, and press the "start/stop" button to switch on the bread machine.
8. When the bread machine beeps, open the lid, then take out the bread basket and lift out the bread.
9. Let it cool for 1 hour, then cut it into fourteen slices and serve.

Nutrition:

Cal 187,

Fat 15.9 g

Protein 6.2 g

Carb 8.8 g

Fiber 5.2 g

Net Carb 3.6 g

129. Pumpkin Bread

Preparation Time: 10 minutes

Cooking time: 4 hours

Servings: 12 slices

Ingredients:

- 2 eggs, pasteurized
- 1 cup / 225 grams almond butter, unsweetened
- 2/3 cup / 130 grams erythritol sweetener
- 2/3 cup / 150 grams pumpkin puree
- 1/8 teaspoon ground cloves
- 1/2 teaspoon ground cinnamon
- 1/8 teaspoon ground ginger
- 1 teaspoon baking powder
- 1/2 teaspoon ground nutmeg

Directions:

1. Gather all the ingredients for the bread and plug in the bread machine having the capacity of 2 pounds of bread recipe.
2. Take a large bowl, crack eggs in it and then beat in the remaining ingredients in it in the order described in the ingredients until incorporated.
3. Add batter into the bread bucket, shut the lid, select the "basic/white" cycle setting and then press the up/down arrow button to adjust baking time according to your bread machine; it will take 3 to 4 hours.
4. Then press the crust button to select light crust if available, and press the "start/stop" button to switch on the bread machine.
5. When the bread machine beeps, open the lid, then take out the bread basket and lift out the bread.
6. Let it cool for 1 hour, then cut it into fourteen slices and serve.

Nutrition:

Cal 150

Fat 12.9 g

Protein 6.7 g

Carb 7 g

Fiber 2 g

Net Carb 5 g

130. Strawberry Bread

Preparation Time: 10 minutes

Cooking time: 4 hours

Servings: 10 slices

Ingredients:

- 5 eggs, pasteurized
- 1 egg white, pasteurized
- 1 ½ teaspoons vanilla extract, unsweetened
- 2 tablespoons heavy whipping cream
- 2 tablespoons sour cream
- 1 cup monk fruit powder
- 1 ½ teaspoons baking powder
- ½ teaspoon salt
- ½ teaspoon cinnamon
- 8 tablespoons butter, melted
- ¾ cup / 100 grams coconut flour
- ¾ cup / 150 grams chopped strawberries

Directions:

1. Gather all the ingredients for the bread and plug in the bread machine having the capacity of 2 pounds of bread recipe.

2. Take a large bowl, crack eggs in it and then beat in egg white, vanilla, heavy cream, sour cream, baking powder, salt, and cinnamon until well combined.
3. Then stir in coconut flour and fold in strawberries until mixed.
4. Add batter into the bread bucket, shut the lid, select the "basic/white" cycle or "low-carb" setting and then press the up/down arrow button to adjust baking time according to your bread machine; it will take 3 to 4 hours.
5. Then press the crust button to select light crust if available, and press the "start/stop" button to switch on the bread machine.
6. When the bread machine beeps, open the lid, then take out the bread basket and lift out the bread.
7. Let it cool for 1 hour, then cut it into fourteen slices and serve.

Nutrition:

Cal 201

Fat 16.4 g

Protein 4.7 g

Carb 6.1 g

Fiber 3 g

Net Carb 3.1 g

131. Blueberry Bread Loaf

Preparation Time: 20 minutes

Cooking time: 65 minutes

Servings: 12

Ingredients:

For the bread dough:

- 10 tbsp. coconut flour

- 9 tbsp. melted butter
- 2/3 cup granulates swerve sweetener
- ½ tsp. baking powder
- 1 tbsp. heavy whipping cream
- 1 ½ tsp. vanilla extract
- ½ tsp. cinnamon
- 3 tbsp. sour cream
- 6 large eggs
- ½ tsp. salt
- ¾ cup blueberries

For the topping:

- 2 tbsp. heavy whipping cream
- 1 tbsp. swerve sweetener
- 1 tsp. melted butter
- 1/8 tsp. vanilla extract
- ¼ tsp. lemon zest

Directions:

1. Gather all the ingredients for the bread and plug in the bread machine having the capacity of 2 pounds of bread recipe.
2. Take a large bowl, crack eggs in it and then beat in cream, butter, and vanilla until combined.
3. Take a separate large bowl, place coconut flour in it, then stir in sweetener and baking powder until mixed and fold in blueberries.
4. Add egg mixture into the bread bucket, top with flour mixture, shut the lid, select the "basic/white" cycle or "low-carb" setting and then press the up/down arrow button to adjust baking time according to your bread machine; it will take 3 to 4 hours.
5. Then press the crust button to select light crust if available, and press the "start/stop" button to switch on the bread machine.

6. When the bread machine beeps, open the lid, then take out the bread basket and lift out the bread.
7. Meanwhile, in a bowl, beat the vanilla extract, butter, heavy whipping cream, lemon zest, and confectioner swerve. Mix until creamy.
8. Then drizzle the icing topping on the bread.
9. Enjoy.

Nutrition:

Calories 155

Fat 13 g

Carb 4 g

Protein 3 g

132. Cranberry And Orange Bread

Preparation Time: 10 minutes

Cooking time: 4 hours

Servings: 12 slices

Ingredients:

- 1 cup / 200 grams chopped cranberries
- 2/3 cup and 3 tablespoons / 175 grams monk fruit powder, divided
- 5 eggs, pasteurized
- 1 egg white, pasteurized
- 2 tablespoons sour cream
- 1 ½ teaspoons orange extract, unsweetened
- 1 teaspoon vanilla extract, unsweetened
- 9 tablespoons butter, grass-fed, unsalted, melted
- 9 tablespoons coconut flour
- 1 ½ teaspoons baking powder

- ¼ teaspoon salt

Directions:

1. Take a small bowl, place cranberries in it, and then stir in 4 tablespoons of monk fruit powder until combined, set aside until required.
2. Gather all the ingredients for the bread and plug in the bread machine having the capacity of 2 pounds of bread recipe.
3. Take a large bowl, crack eggs in it, beat in remaining ingredients in it in the order described in the ingredients until incorporated, and then fold in cranberries until just mixed.
4. Add batter into the bread bucket, shut the lid, select the "basic/white" cycle or "low-carb" setting and then press the up/down arrow button to adjust baking time according to your bread machine; it will take 3 to 4 hours.
5. Then press the crust button to select light crust if available, and press the "start/stop" button to switch on the bread machine.
6. When the bread machine beeps, open the lid, then take out the bread basket and lift out the bread.
7. Let it cool for 1 hour, then cut it into fourteen slices and serve.

Nutrition:

Cal 149,

Fat 13.1 g

Protein 3.9 g

Carb 4 g

Fiber 1.5 g

Net Carb 2.5 g

133. Chocolate Chip Beloved Bread

Preparation Time: 10 minutes

Cooking time: 3 hours

Servings: 12 slices/2lbs

Ingredients:

- 1/3 cup brown sugar
- 2 tbsps. butter softened
- cup warm milk,
- 1 large pc Egg
- cups Bread flour
- 1 ½ tsps. Salt
- 1 ½ tsps. Bread machine yeast
- 1/3 cup Cocoa powder
- 3/4 cup Chocolate chips

Directions:

1. Add all the ingredients in the bread machine's pan in the manufacturer's recommended order (except 50% chocolate chips).
2. Put the 50% chocolate chips in the fruit and nut dispenser. If you lack a fruit and nut dispenser, you can add nuts directly to the bread.
3. Set the program of your bread machine to Basic/White Bread and set crust type to Light 2-pound loaf and press START.
4. When ready, allow about 10 minutes to cool and serve.
5. Wrap in plastic wrap after completely cooled. Enjoy!

Nutrition:

Calories: 184

Carbs: 30.6g

Fat: 5.2g

Protein: 4.8g

134. Poppy Seed And Prune Bread

Preparation Time: 10 minutes

Cooking time: 58 minutes

Servings: 12 slices

Ingredients:

- 1/2 cup Prunes, finely chopped
- 1 tsp. Vanilla extract
- ½ tsp. of Salt
- 2 tsp. Baking powder
- 1 tbsp. Poppy seeds
- 1 tbsp. grated orange peel
- 1/2 cup Sugar
- 1 1/2 cups all-purpose flour
- 1/3 cup unsalted butter, softened
- 2 large eggs, beaten
- ½ cup (120ml) lukewarm milk

Directions:

1. Put the following ingredients into a mixing bowl in this order: milk, beaten eggs, butter, flour, sugar, poppy seeds, orange peel, baking powder, salt, and vanilla extract. Mix until combined. Transfer to a bread pan.
2. Choose the Quick bread or Express Bake setting. Press START.
3. Wait for the add ingredient beep before adding the prunes.
4. Once done, transfer the baked bread to a wire rack and leave for 20 minutes to cool before slicing.
5. Enjoy!

Nutrition:

Calories: 232

Carbs: 20.5g

Fat: 10g

Protein: 13g

135. Blessed Bread

Preparation Time: 15 minutes

Cooking time: 3 hours

Servings: 12 slices

Ingredients:

- 2/3 cup of walnuts, chopped
- 2¼ tsps. of Bread machine yeast
- 4 cups of bread flour
- 1½ cups Instant or regular oatmeal
- 1 tsp. of Salt
- ¾ tsp. Lemon extract
- 6 tbsps. (88ml)   Maple syrup
- 6 tbsps. (88ml)   Vegetable oil
- 11/3 cups (320ml) warm water

Directions:

1. Group all the ingredients (except the walnuts) in your bread machine pan according to the manufacturer's suggestion. I start with liquids and then add dry ingredients.
2. I add yeast at the end, form a well on top of the dry ingredients, and put the yeast on the hole.
3. Snap the pan in the chamber and close the lid. Put the walnuts in the fruit and nut dispenser. If you lack a fruit and nut dispenser, you can add walnuts directly to the bread pan when you hear the added ingredient beep.
4. Choose the Basic setting and your preferred crust color. Press START.
5. Put the baked bread on a wire rack and allow cooling before slicing.

6. Enjoy!

Nutrition:

Calories: 200

Carbs: 2g

Fat: 9g

Protein: 13g

136. Fast And Fabulous

Preparation Time: 10 minutes

Cooking time: 2 hours 10 minutes

Servings: 12 slices

Ingredients:

- 1 cup (240ml) warm milk
- 3 tbsps. Molasses
- 1 large Egg
- 2 tbsps. Margarine
- ¾ tsp. Salt
- ¼ tsp. Ground cloves -
- ½ tsp. Ground cinnamon -
- 3/4 tsp. Ground ginger -
- 2 tsps.   Bread machine yeast
- 2 tbsps. Brown sugar
- 31/3 cups Bread flour

Directions:

1. Add all the ingredients in the bread machine's pan in the manufacturer's recommended order (combine the milk and egg before adding to the pan).
2. Select Rapid Bake setting for a 2-pound loaf.

3. Once done, carefully transfer bread to a wire rack and leave to cool for 20 minutes.
4. Slice and serve.
5. Enjoy!

Nutrition:

Calories: 200

Carbs: 2g

Fat: 9g

Protein: 13g

137. Regal Raisin Bread

Preparation Time: 10 minutes

Cooking time: 3 hours

Servings: 12 slices

Ingredients:

- 1 cup Raisins
- 2 ¼ tsps. Active dry yeast
- 1 ½ tsps. Ground Cinnamon
- 2 tbsps. Dry milk
- 3 tbsps. Sugar
- 4 cups Bread flour
- 1 ½ tsps. Salt
- 2 tbsp. butter softened
- 1 ¼ cups (300ml) warm water -

Directions:

1. Put all the liquid ingredients in the pan.
2. Add all the dry ingredients, in the pan, except the yeast and raisins.

3. Form a well on top of the dry ingredients and put the yeast on the hole.
4. Snap the pan in the chamber and close the lid.
5. Choose the Basic setting and your preferred crust color. Press START.
6. Wait for the add ingredient beep before raising the lid. Gradually sprinkle the raisins until they're combined with the dough.
7. Let it cool for 1 hour, then cut it into fourteen slices and serve.
8. Enjoy!

Nutrition:

Calories: 180

Carbs: 38g

Fat: 2g

Protein: 4g

138. Holiday Holler

Preparation Time: 10 minutes

Cooking Time: 3 hours 5 minutes

Servings: 16 slices

Ingredients:

- 3 tsp. Bread machine yeast
- 3¼ cups Bread flour
- 1 tsp. Salt
- 1 tsp. Anise seed -
- 1½ tsps. dried orange peel
- ¼ cup Candied lemon peel, diced
- ¼ cup Candied cherries, diced
- ½ cup Mixed candied fruits, diced
- 1/3 cup Sugar

- 1/3 cup butter, cubed
- 2/3 cup (160ml) warm milk
- 2 large pc. Eggs

Directions:

1. Group all the ingredients in your bread machine pan according to the manufacturer's directions, except pine nuts).
2. Secure the pan into the chamber and close the lid.
3. Put the pine nuts in the fruit and nut dispenser. If you lack a fruit and nut dispenser, you can add nuts directly into the bread pan when you hear the added ingredient beep.
4. Turn the machine on. Press the Sweet setting and your chosen crust color. Press START.
5. Once done baking, transfer the bread to a wire rack to cool.
6. Enjoy!

Nutrition:

Calories: 190

Carbs: 23g

Fat: 9g

Protein: 1g

139. Charming Challah

Preparation Time: 10 minutes

Cooking time: 3 hours

Servings: 10 slices

Ingredients:

- ¾ cup (180ml)   Milk
- 2 pcs. Eggs

- 3 tbsps. Margarine
- ¼ cup   Sugar
- 1½ tsps. Salt
- 1½ tsps. Active dry yeast

Directions:

1. Group all of the ingredients to your bread machine, carefully following the instructions from the manufacturer.
2. Set the program of your bread machine to Basic/White Bread and set crust type to Light.
3. Press START.
4. Wait until the cycle completes.
5. Let it cool for 1 hour, then cut it into fourteen slices and serve.
6. Shake the bucket to remove the loaf.
7. Slice, and serve. Enjoy!

Nutrition:

Calories: 184

Carbs: 30g

Fat: 4g

Protein: 6g

140. Chocolate Bread With Hazelnuts

Preparation Time: 15 minutes

Cooking time: 2 hours 50 minutes

Servings: 10 slices

Ingredients:

- ½ cup Hazelnuts, chopped
- 2 tsps. Bread machine yeast

- 4 cups   Bread flour Salt
- ½ cup Sugar
- 1/3 cup unsweetened cocoa powder
- 2 tbsps. butter softened
- ¾ cup (180ml) warm water
- 2 Eggs large.

Directions:

1. Group all the ingredients in your bread machine pan according to the manufacturer's advice (except hazelnuts).
2. Place the hazelnuts in the fruit and nut dispenser. If you lack a fruit and nut dispenser, you can add nuts directly to the bread pan when you hear the added ingredient beep.
3. Choose the Sweet setting and your preferred crust color. Press START.
4. Let it cool for 1 hour, then cut it into fourteen slices and serve.

Nutrition:

Calories: 226

Carbs: 21g

Fat: 15g

Protein: 4g

Chapter 13. Whole Wheat Bread

141. Whole Wheat Peanut Butter And Jelly Bread

Preparation Time: 10m

Cooking time: 2h50m

Servings: 12

Ingredients:

- 10 ounce. water
- 1/2 cup peanut butter
- 1/2 cup strawberry jelly
- 1 1/2 tbsps. light brown sugar
- 1/2 tsp. salt
- 3/4 tsp. baking soda
- 3/4 tsp. baking powder
- 3 tbsps. vital wheat gluten
- 3 1/3 cups whole wheat flour
- 1 tbsp. whole wheat flour
- 1 1/2 tsps. active dry yeast

Directions:

1. Into the bread machine pan, add the following in this order; sugar baking powder peanut butter, jelly, brown water, salt, baking soda, gluten, 3 1/3 cups plus 1 tbsp.: whole wheat flour, and yeast.
2. Choose 1 1/2 Pound Loaf, Medium Crust, Wheat cycle, and then start the machine.

Nutrition:

Calories: 230

Total Carbohydrate: 38.6 g

Cholesterol: 0 mg

Total Fat: 6.1 g

Protein: 8.7 g

Sodium: 259 mg

142. Bread Machine Ezekiel Bread

Preparation Time: 10 minutes

Cooking time: 3 hours

Servings: 10 slices

Ingredients:

- 1/2 cup milk
- 1/2 cup water
- 1 egg
- 2 1/2 tbsps. olive oil, divided
- 1 tbsp. honey
- 1 tbsp. dry black beans
- 1 tbsp. dry lentils
- 1 tbsp. dry kidney beans
- 1 tbsp. barley
- 1 cup unbleached all-purpose flour
- 1 cup whole wheat flour
- 1/4 cup millet flour
- 1/4 cup rye flour
- 1/4 cup cracked wheat
- 2 tbsps. wheat germ
- 1 tsp. salt
- 2 tsps. yeast

Directions:

1. Using a safe glass measuring cup, add water and milk, and then heat for about 35 seconds in the microwave.
2. Using a coffee grinder, grind the barley, kidney beans, black beans, and lentils until fine.
3. Use a cloth to cover and leave to rise.
4. Remove the cover from the dough and then bake for 10 minutes in the oven.
5. Let it cool then, slice.

Nutrition:

Calories: 192;

Total Carbohydrate: 31.5 g

Cholesterol: 20 mg

Total Fat: 5 g

Protein: 6.6 g

Sodium: 247 mg

143. Bread Machine Honey-Oat-Wheat Bread

Preparation Time: 10m

Cooking time: 3h15m

Servings: 12

Ingredients:

- 2 1/2 tsps. active dry yeast
- 2 tbsps. sugar
- 1 1/2 cups warm water

- 3 cups all-purpose flour
- 1 cup whole wheat flour
- 1 cup rolled oats
- 3 tbsps. powdered milk
- 1 tsp. salt
- 1/4 cup honey
- 1/4 cup vegetable oil
- 3 tbsps. butter softened
- cooking spray

Directions:

1. Into the pan of a bread machine, put the yeast, sugar, and water. Let yeast dissolve and foam for approximately 10 minutes. In a bowl, mix the all-purpose flour, powdered milk, whole wheat flour, salt, and rolled oats. Reserve. Pour the butter, honey, and vegetable oil into the yeast mixture. Then add the flour mixture on top.
2. Choose the Dough cycle and then push the start button. Let the bread machine to finish the cycle, approximately 1 1/2 hours.
3. Bake for about 40 minutes and let it cool, then slice.

Nutrition:

Calories: 281

Total Carbohydrate: 44.7 g

Cholesterol: 10 mg

Total Fat: 8.9 g

Protein: 6.4 g

Sodium: 225 mg

144. Butter Honey Wheat Bread

Preparation Time: 5m

Cooking time: 3h5m

Servings: 12

Ingredients:

- 1 cup of water
- 2 tbsps. margarine
- 2 tbsps. honey
- 2 cups bread flour
- 1/2 cup whole wheat flour
- 1/3 cup dry milk powder
- 1 tsp. salt
- 1 (.25 ounce.) package active dry yeast

Directions:

1. Follow the order of putting the ingredients into the bread machine recommended by the manufacturer.
2. Run the bread machine for a large loaf (1-1/2 lb.) on a Wheat setting.

Nutrition:

Calories: 57 calories;

Total Carbohydrate: 8.5 g

Cholesterol: 1 mg

Total Fat: 1.9 g

Protein: 2.1 g

Sodium: 234 mg

145. Buttermilk Bread I

Preparation Time: 15 minutes

Cooking time: 2 hours 50 minutes

Servings: 12

Ingredients:

- 1 1/2 cups buttermilk
- 1 1/2 tbsps. margarine
- 2 tbsps. white sugar
- 1 tsp. salt
- 3 cups bread flour
- 1 1/3 cups whole wheat flour
- 2 1/4 tsps. active dry yeast

Directions:

1. Into the bread machine pan, add buttermilk, butter or margarine, sugar, salt, flour, whole wheat flour, and yeast in that order.
2. Bake using the White Bread setting. Then transfer onto wire racks to cool prior to slicing.

Nutrition:

Calories: 80

Total Carbohydrate: 13.5 g

Cholesterol: 1 mg

Total Fat: 1.9 g

Protein: 3.1 g

Sodium: 243 mg

146. Buttermilk Wheat Bread

Servings: 12

Preparation Time: 8m

Cooking time: 6h8m

Ingredients:

- 1 1/2 cups buttermilk
- 1 1/2 tbsps. butter, melted
- 2 tbsps. white sugar
- 3/4 tsp. salt
- 3 cups all-purpose flour
- 1/3 cup whole wheat flour
- 1 1/2 tsps. active dry yeast

Directions:

1. In the bread machine pan, measure all ingredients in the order the manufacturer recommended. Set the machine to the Basic White Bread setting.
2. Start the machine.
3. After a few minutes, add more buttermilk if the ingredients do not form a ball, or if it is too loose, put a handful of flour.

Nutrition:

Calories: 160 calories;

Total Carbohydrate: 30 g

Cholesterol: 5 mg

Total Fat: 2.1 g

Protein: 4.9 g

Sodium: 189 mg

147. Ricotta & Chive Loaf

Preparation Time: 30-45 minutes

Cooking Time: 30-45 minutes

Servings: 1 loaf

Ingredients:

- 1/3 cup whole ricotta cheese
- 1 cup lukewarm water
- 1½ teaspoons salt
- 1 tablespoon granulated sugar
- ½ cups bread flour
- ½ cup chopped chives
- 2½ teaspoons instant yeast

Directions:

1. Add all of the ingredients to your bread machine, carefully following the instructions of the manufacturer (except dried fruits).
2. Set the program of your bread machine to Basic/White Bread and set crust type to Light.
3. Press START.
4. Once the machine beeps, add fruits.
5. Wait until the cycle completes.
6. Once the loaf is ready, take the bucket out and let the loaf cool for 5 minutes.
7. Gently shake the bucket to remove the loaf.
8. Transfer to a cooling rack, slice, and serve.

9. Enjoy!

Nutrition:

Calories: 281

Total Carbohydrate: 44.7 g

Cholesterol: 10 mg

Total Fat: 8.9 g

Protein: 6.4 g

Sodium: 225 mg

148. Crunchy Honey Wheat Bread

Preparation Time: 15 minutes

Cooking time: 2 hours 50 minutes

Servings: 12

Ingredients:

- 1 1/4 cups warm water
- 2 tbsps. vegetable oil
- 3 tbsps. honey
- 1 1/2 tsps. salt
- 2 cups bread flour
- 1 1/2 cups whole wheat flour
- 1 tbsp. vital wheat gluten
- 1/2 cup granola
- 1 (.25 oz.) package active dry yeast

Directions:

1. Put the ingredients into the pan of the bread machine following the order recommended by the manufacturer.
2. Choose the Whole Wheat setting or the Dough cycle on the machine. Press the Start button.
3. Baking the bread in the oven: Choose the Dough cycle or the Manual cycle on the bread machine. Once the machine has finished the whole cycle, form the dough and put it into a loaf pan that is greased. Let it rise in volume in a warm place until it becomes double its size. Put in the preheated 350°F (175°C) oven and bake for 35-45 minutes or until a poked thermometer in the middle of the loaf indicates 200°F (95°C).

Nutrition:

Calories: 199 calories;

Total Carbohydrate: 34.9 g

Cholesterol: 0 mg

Total Fat: 4.2 g

Protein: 6.2 g

Sodium: 294 mg

149. Easy Whole Wheat Bread

Preparation Time: 10m

Cooking time: 3h10m

Servings: 12

Ingredients:

- 3/4 cup of warm water

- 1 tbsp. powdered egg substitute (optional)
- 2 tbsps. vegetable oil
- 2 tbsps. sugar
- 1 tsp. salt
- 1 cup bread flour
- 1 cup whole wheat flour
- 1 tsp. rapid rise yeast

Directions:

1. Start by dissolving the egg substitute in warm water. Into the bread machine pan, add all ingredients following the order prescribed on the machine's manual. Use a whole-wheat cycle and regular bake time and start the machine.
2. Check the way the dough is kneading when five minutes elapse because you may need to add either one tbsp. of water or one tbsp. of flour, but it depends on the consistency. When the bread is done, cool it on a wire rack prior to slicing.

Nutrition:

Calories: 65 calories;

Total Carbohydrate: 9.6 g

Cholesterol: 0 mg

Total Fat: 2.5 g

Protein: 1.7 g

Sodium: 198 mg

150. Essene Bread For The Bread Machine

Preparation Time: 1h30m

Cooking time: 3days11h20m

Servings: 15

Ingredients:

- 1/2 cup sprouted wheat berries, ground
- 3/4 cup buttermilk
- 1 egg
- 2 tbsps. maple syrup
- 1/2 tsp. salt
- 1/3 tsp. baking soda
- 2 tbsps. vital wheat gluten
- 2 1/4 cups whole wheat flour
- 1 1/2 tsps. active dry yeast

Directions:

1. Prepare this bread a couple of days in advance if you plan to make it; start by washing 1/2 cup of the raw wheat berries in cool water, then drain it. In a big bowl, let the rinsed berries soak in cool water. Use a cloth or a plate to cover the berries and let it soak at standard room temperature for about 12 hours or throughout the night. The berries will absorb a good amount of water. Use a colander to drain the soaked berries and use a plate to cover the colander to keep the berries from dehydrating; place it in an area without light. Wash the berries about thrice a day, and soon you'll see them produce shoots. After a few days, the sprouts will attain their optimal length, which is about 1/4 inch in size. Drain off the berry sprouts and use a food processor or a blender to crush the sprouts.
2. In the bread machine pan, put in the ingredients following the order suggested by the manufacturer. Choose the Whole Wheat and the Medium Crust setting on the machine and press the Start button to run the machine.
3. If the Raisin cycle is available on the bread machine used, put in the sprouts at the machine's signal to keep the sprouts intact. If there's no Raisin cycle

available in the bread machine used, the texture of the bread may be a bit pulpy.

Nutrition:

Calories: 104;

Total Carbohydrate: 20.6 g

Cholesterol: 13 mg

Total Fat: 0.9 g

Protein: 4.9 g

Sodium: 124 mg

151. Hot Buttered Rum Bread

Preparation Time: 10 minutes

Cooking Time: 20-30 minutes

Servings: 1 loaf

Ingredients:

- ½ cup minus 1 tablespoon water, at 80°F to 90°F
- 2 egg, at room temperature
- 2 tablespoons butter, melted and cooled
- 1 tablespoon sugar
- 2 teaspoons rum extract
- ¾ teaspoon salt
- ⅔ teaspoon ground cinnamon
- ¼ teaspoon ground nutmeg
- 2 cups white bread flour
- ⅓ teaspoon bread machine

Directions:

1. Add all of the ingredients to your device.
2. Set the program of your bread machine to Basic/White Bread and set crust type to Medium.
3. Press START.
4. Wait until the cycle completes.
5. Once the loaf is ready, take the bucket out and let the loaf cool for a while.
6. Shake the bucket gently to remove the loaf.
7. Enjoy!

Nutrition:

Calories: 161

Total Fat: 4g

Saturated Fat: 2g

Carbohydrates: 27g

Fiber: 1g

Sodium: 271mg

Protein: 4g

152. Honey-Flavored Bread

Preparation Time: 30-45 minutes

Cooking Time: 30-45 minutes

Servings: Makes 1 loaf

Ingredients:

- 2¼ cups white flour

- ¼ cup rye flour
- 2 cup of water
- 2 whole egg, beaten
- 1 tablespoon vegetable oil
- 1 teaspoon salt
- 1½ tablespoons honey
- 1 teaspoon dry yeast

Directions:

1. Group all of the ingredients to your device, carefully following the instructions of the manufacturer.
2. Set the program of your bread machine to Basic/White Bread and set crust type to Medium.
3. Press START.
4. Wait until the cycle completes.
5. Once the loaf is ready, take the bucket out and let it cool for 5 minutes.
6. Slice, and serve.

Nutrition:

Total Carbs: 33g

Fiber: 1g

Protein: 6g

Fat: 3g,

Calories: 177

153. Pantone Bread

Preparation Time: 10 minutes

Cooking Time: 20-30 minutes

Servings: Makes 1 loaf

Ingredients:

- ¾ cup milk, at 80°F to 90°F
- ¼ cup melted butter, cooled
- 2 eggs, at room temperature
- 2 teaspoons pure vanilla extract
- 2 tablespoons sugar
- 1½ teaspoons salt
- 3¼ cups white bread flour
- 2 teaspoons bread machine or instant yeast
- ¼ cup candied lemon peel
- ¼ cup candied orange peel

Directions:

1. Place the ingredients, except the candied fruit peel, in your bread machine as recommended by the manufacturer.
2. Program the machine for Sweet bread, select light or medium crust, and press Start.
3. When the machine signals, add the peel, or place in the nut/raisin hopper and let the machine add the peel automatically.
4. When the loaf is done, remove the bucket from the machine.
5. Let the loaf cool for 5 minutes.
6. Gently shake the bucket to remove the loaf, and turn it out onto a rack to cool.

Nutrition:

Calories: 104;

Total Carbohydrate: 20.6 g

Cholesterol: 13 mg

Total Fat: 0.9 g

Protein: 4.9 g

Sodium: 124 mg

154. Delicious Flax Honey Loaf

Preparation Time: 30-45 minutes

Cooking Time: 30-45 minutes

Servings: 1 loaf

Ingredients:

- ¾ cup milk, at room temperature
- 1 tablespoon melted butter
- 1 tablespoon honey
- ¾ teaspoon salt
- tablespoons flaxseeds
- cups white bread flour
- ¾ teaspoon bread machine yeast

Directions:

1. Sift both types of flour in a bowl and mix.
2. Group all of the ingredients to your device.
3. Set the program of your bread machine to Basic/White Bread and set crust type to Medium.

4. Press START.
5. Wait until the cycle completes.
6. Once the loaf is ready, take the bucket out and let the loaf cool for 5 minutes.
7. Shake the bucket to remove the loaf.
8. Transfer to a cooling plate, slice, and serve.

Nutrition:

Total Carbs: 28g

Fiber: 1g

Protein: 6g

Fat: 3g,

Calories: 158

155. Raisin Bran Bread

Preparation Time: 10 minutes

Cooking Time: 20-25 minutes

Servings: 1 loaf

Ingredients:

- ¾ cup of milk
- 1½ tablespoons melted butter, cooled
- 2 tablespoons sugar
- ½ teaspoon salt
- ¼ cup wheat bran
- 1¾ cups white bread flour
- 1 teaspoon bread machine or instant yeast
- ½ cup raisins

Directions:

1. Place the ingredients, except the raisins.
2. Set the device for Basic/White bread, select light or medium crust, and press Start.
3. Add the raisins, or put them in the nut/raisin hopper and let your machine add them automatically.
4. When the loaf is processed, remove the bucket from the device.
5. Gently shake the bucket. Let it cool, and slice.

Nutrition:

Calories: 173

Total Fat: 3g

Saturated Fat: 2g

Carbohydrates: 34g

Fiber: 2g

Sodium: 317mg

Protein: 4g

156. Oat Bran Molasses Bread

Preparation Time: 10 minutes

Cooking Time: 20-30 minutes

Servings: 1 loaf

Ingredients:

- ¾ cup of water
- 2¼ tablespoons melted butter, cooled

- 3 tablespoons blackstrap molasses
- ⅓ teaspoon salt
- ¼ teaspoon ground nutmeg
- ¾ cup oat bran
- 2¼ cups whole-wheat bread flour
- 1⅔ teaspoons bread machine

Directions:

1. Group the ingredients in your device.
2. Set the machine for Whole-Wheat/Whole-Grain bread, select light or medium crust, and press Start.
3. When the loaf is processed, remove the bucket from the machine.
4. Let the loaf cool for a while.
5. Slice and serve.

Nutrition:

Calories: 137

Total Fat: 3g

Saturated Fat: 2g

Carbohydrates: 25g

Fiber: 1g

Sodium: 112mg

Protein: 3g

157. Bran Bread

Preparation Time: 30-45 minutes

Cooking Time: 30-45 minutes

Servings: 1 loaf

Ingredients:

- 2 ½ cups (320 g) all-purpose flour, sifted
- 2 whole egg
- ¾ cup (40 g) bran
- 1 cup (240 ml) lukewarm water
- 1 tablespoon sunflower oil
- 1 teaspoon brown sugar
- 1 teaspoon of sea salt
- 1 teaspoon active dry yeast

Directions:

1. Prepare all of the ingredients for your bread and measuring means (a cup, a spoon, kitchen scales).
2. Carefully measure the ingredients into the pan.
3. Group all of the ingredients into the device in the right order, following the manual for your bread machine.
4. Close the cover.
5. Select the program of your bread machine to FRENCH BREAD and choose the crust color to MEDIUM.
6. Press START.
7. Wait until the program completes.
8. When done, take the bucket out and let it cool for 5-10 minutes.
9. Shake the loaf from the pan and let cool for 30 minutes on a cooling rack.
10. Slice, serve, and enjoy the taste of fragrant homemade bread.

Nutrition:

Calories 307

Total Fat 5.1g

Saturated Fat 0.9g

Cholesterol 33g

Sodium 480mg

Total Carbohydrate 54g

Dietary Fiber 7.9g

Total Sugars 1.8g

Protein 10.2g

158. Whole-Wheat Challah

Preparation Time: 10 minutes

Cooking Time: 20-30 minutes

Servings: 1 loaf

Ingredients:

- ½ cup of water
- ¼ cup melted butter cooled
- 2 egg, at room temperature
- ½ teaspoon salt
- 1 tablespoon sugar
- ¾ cup whole-wheat flour
- 1¼ cups white bread flour
- 1⅛ teaspoon bread machine

Directions:

1. Group all of the ingredients to your device.
2. Set the program of your bread machine to Basic/White Bread and set crust type to Medium.
3. Press START.

4. Wait until the cycle completes.
5. Once the loaf is ready, take the bucket out and let the loaf cool for 5 minutes.
6. Shake the bucket gently to remove the loaf.
7. Slice, and serve.

Nutrition:

Calories: 183

Total Fat: 6g

Saturated Fat: 4g

Carbohydrates: 27g fiber: 1g

Sodium: 339mg

Protein: 5g

159. Whole-Wheat Sourdough Bread

Preparation Time: 10 minutes

Cooking Time: 20-30 minutes

Servings: 1 loaf

Ingredients:

- ¾ cup of water
- ¾ cup plus 2 tablespoons No-Yeast Whole-Wheat Sourdough Starter (here), fed, active, and at room temperature
- 2 tablespoons melted butter, cooled
- 1 tablespoon sugar
- 1½ teaspoons salt
- 4 cups whole-wheat flour
- 1¾ teaspoons bread machine

Directions:

1. Group all of the ingredients to your device.
2. Set the program of your bread machine to Basic/White Bread and set crust type to Medium.
3. Press START.
4. Wait until the cycle completes.
5. Once the loaf is ready, take the bucket out and let the loaf cool for 5 minutes.
6. Shake the bucket gently to remove the loaf.
7. Slice, and serve.

Nutrition:

Calories: 155

Total Fat: 2g

Saturated Fat: 1g

Carbohydrates: 29g

Fiber: 1g

Sodium: 305mg

Protein: 4g

160. Faithful Italian Semolina Bread

Preparation Time: 30-45 minutes

Cooking Time: 30-45 minutes

Servings: 1 loaf

Ingredients:

- 2½ tablespoons butter

- 2½ teaspoons sugar
- 2¼ cups flour
- ⅓ cups semolina
- 1½ teaspoons dry yeast
- 1 cup of water
- 1 teaspoon salt

Directions:

1. Group all of the ingredients to your device
2. Set the program of your bread machine to Italian Bread/Sandwich mode and set crust type to Medium.
3. Press START.
4. Wait until the cycle completes.
5. Once the loaf is ready, take the bucket out and let the loaf cool for a while.
6. Shake the bucket gently to remove the loaf.
7. Slice, and serve.

Nutrition:

Total Carbs: 45g

Fiber: 1g

Protein: 7g

Fat: 10g

Calories: 302

Conclusion

A bread machine is the best way to bake bread. By adding all the ingredients to the bread pan without touching anything, you can put a piece of bread in your bread machine. Make baking a hobby! Getting creative is not a difficult task when you learn the techniques of bread making. The ease and convenience of baking bread in your bread machine is worth the bother. Baking bread is a great activity for people that are not particularly strong and also a good way to use up old bread. You don't have to make bread; you can bake bread for your family using your bread machine.

Baking bread in a bread maker can take just minutes to prepare! You'll find that it's quite simple to make sure your baking pan bread machine bread. You need to have a roomy bread machine pan. You must also have specific bread baking recipes for your family and the food supply to use for you.

The right technique is essential if you want good bread and to become the queen or king of the dinner table! You shouldn't be afraid to try some new recipes. Most bread machine bakers will shun whole-wheat breads; avoid them at all costs. Why? Whole wheat breads are stickier than white breads and have a tendency to clog you.

It's easy to keep your bread machine pan clean with a few simple tips. First, clean the bread machine pan immediately after using it. By leaving the dough to harden in the pan, you make it harder to clean the pan. Some people add salt to their bread recipes to make the crust crispier; salty crusts may take longer to clean. Sometimes will find that the crusts begin to darken and brown as they heat up. These dark crusts can also dull the pan and result in less capacity. Lastly, avoid over toasting your bread. It's okay to make a grilled cheese request by putting the bread pan into the toaster once in a while just to keep it clean.

A good way to tell if the bread is done is to check on it every 10 minutes after the first hour. Gently pry open the lid.

Baking bread in a bread-machine allows you to combine all the ingredients to the bread machine pan without using a separate pan. This will save you an awful lot of time and effort when you want to bake bread. Some food saves time and effort better than others. Bread is one that saves you time but want you to have it still. The Bread machine is not only for making quick breads and pastries. It is also a great choice for beginners who want to make homemade bread. Fresh bread, homemade daily, is not only good-tasting but it can also be good for you. It unfailingly lures everyone who enters the house for a taste. Baking bread in a bread machine is an excellent way to make sure that you always have quality bread on hand without the drudgery of conventional baking.

Baking bread in a bread machine can be a fun way to spend time in the kitchen, and it can be a very rewarding hobby or even a business to make fresh bread for friends and family. You may also consider making all your bread recipes from a bread machine if you don't have the time to bake from scratch. Baking bread in a bread machine can surely become a very rewarding hobby or way to make extra cash.

At the end of the day, the taste of the bread is the same no matter what machine. Try this fresh bread recipe from a bread machine and you will be amazed.

Enjoying baking fresh bread at home!